Dyslexia and Alternative Therapies

Dyslexia and Alternative Therapies

Maria Chivers

Jessica Kingsley Publishers
London and Philadelphia

First published in 2006
by Jessica Kingsley Publishers
116 Pentonville Road
London N1 9JB, UK
and
400 Market Street, Suite 400
Philadelphia, PA 19106, USA

www.jkp.com

Library of Congress Cataloging in Publication Data

Chivers, Maria.
  Dyslexia and alternative therapies / Maria Chivers.
      p. cm.
  Includes bibliographical references and index.
  ISBN-13: 978-1-84310-378-3 (pbk.)
  ISBN-10: 1-84310-378-8 (pbk.)
   1. Dyslexia--Alternative treatment. 2. Learning disabilities--Alternative treatment. 3. Dyslexic children. I.
Title.
  RJ496.A5C473 2006
  616.85'5306--dc22

                                                    2006012372

British Library Cataloguing in Publication Data
A CIP catalogue record for this book is available from the British Library

ISBN-13: 978 1 84310 378 3
ISBN-10: 1 84310 378 8

Printed and bound in the United States
by Thomson-Shore, Inc.

To Chris with love

ACKNOWLEDGEMENTS

I would like to express my thanks to the specialists who have kindly contributed to this book: Keith Holland, Chris Vickers, David Mulhall, Angela Lawrence, and to the British Dyslexia Association, for their help over the years, to me personally and professionally.

A NOTE TO THE READER

The material in this book is for informational purposes only. It is not intended to serve as a prescription for you or to replace the advice of your medical doctor. Please discuss all aspects of the complementary or alternative therapy with your physician before beginning any programme.

This book does not set out to promote or guarantee the effectiveness of any of the therapies listed, but to offer useful information for anyone wanting to find out more about alternative therapies, particularly those therapies thought to be effective for use with people with dyslexia.

I have used he throughout the book for ease of reading.

CONTENTS

The doctor of the future will give no medicine,
but will interest his patients in the care of the human frame,
in diet and in the cause and prevention of diseases.

Thomas Edison
(1847–1931)

INTRODUCTION

If you are interested in what alternative therapies have to offer people with dyslexia, ADHD or other learning difficulties, whether a parent, teacher or other professional, this book will offer accessible, helpful advice. I have been working in the education field for over 20 years, and in particular my work at the Swindon Dyslexia Centre has included dealing with thousands of people who were desperately seeking the 'cure' for dyslexia.

For many years dyslexia has been under the scrutiny of many different specialists including audiologists, optometrists, dieticians, linguists, psychologists and more recently complementary and alternative therapists. The result has been a wealth of information, but where do you start? In this book I have looked at over 50 complementary or alternative therapies that have at some time claimed to help, alleviate or even 'cure' dyslexia, ADHD and other specific learning difficulties (besides many other conditions). Entire books have been dedicated to individual therapies. I only intend to give you a 'flavour' of each here. Some of these therapies are very new while others, like Ayurveda, have been around for over 5000 years.

Whilst I have tried to put therapies in the relevant sections, it is sometimes difficult to determine where one method ends and another begins, but the structure used aims to be as helpful and clear as possible. There are now so many 'therapies' that claim to be cure-alls – from fish oils to massage. Within the field of dyslexia, there are a number of people who are suspicious about the merits of 'alternative therapies', just as there are in any other field, and my intention here is not to make the case for complementary medicine – just to offer information and reliable guidance, with evidence where it is available. One thing that is clear is that good old tried and tested teaching methods should not be replaced, and that alternative approaches should be treated as complementary.

This book is written in an easy-to-follow format, with useful addresses relating to each chapter listed at the back of the book to point you in the right direction to get appropriate help. After reading this book you will be in a better position to judge for yourself the merits of acupuncture, coloured glasses, exercises and audio therapies, to name but a few. You may find some of the methods appear a little unorthodox but it will pay dividends to keep an open mind.

Chapter 1

ALTERNATIVE THERAPIES

Complementary and alternative medicine, or CAM as it is often called, covers a range of therapies including herbal medicines, Ayurveda, homeopathy, chiropractic, and many others. Alternative therapy is one of the fastest growing markets in the developed world. Its profile has been helped by the support of prominent people such as Prince Charles and Gwyneth Paltrow and the growing acceptance of the medical establishment. Over a third of people in the United States use alternative therapies and many US health companies offer discounts for certain therapies. This market is said to be worth over $30 billion, whilst a UK-based survey (Ernst and White 2000) revealed Britons spend approximately £1.6 billion a year, which is also predicted to rise substantially as more and more people come to realize the importance of taking responsibility for promoting and maintaining their own health.

It was not so many years ago that chiropractic was considered an alternative therapy, but is now seen as mainstream. A chiropractor may take a couple of hours to alleviate a person's back problem at just a fraction of what back surgery may cost.

The difference between traditional medicine – where the doctor heals the symptoms only – and CAM is that the latter has a focus on respect for the human body and its innate healing abilities. CAM assists the natural healing wisdom of the body through natural approaches, thereby treating the whole person rather than just the presenting problems.

Throughout the media – television, radio, newspapers – you come across alternative therapies that claim to cure dyslexia and specific learning difficulties (SpLDs), amongst other conditions. It should be made clear that dyslexia is not a disease and therefore cannot be 'cured' – despite what some therapists may claim. Also, each dyslexic learner is different. No single method will suit them all because dyslexia encompasses myriad difficulties, including reading, spelling, numeracy, memory problems, organization and, perhaps most important of all, self-esteem.

Only you can look at the therapies and decide whether to 'give them a go' or if you may think they are just a lot of 'hype'. I cannot make up your mind, one way or another, but sometimes it is good to keep an open mind.

Do complementary and alternative therapies work?

Many alternative therapies have not been evaluated in scientific studies. There is often little or no evidence as to their safety or effectiveness and whether they work for particular diseases or medical conditions. Many people have no doubt that alternative therapies definitely work, but it is sometimes difficult to separate the success of a specific treatment from the natural ups and downs of illness or from the benefits of an individual's positive attitude. For instance, research has shown that many things can influence performance:

- *Placebo effects* – in placebo effects, illnesses can be 'cured' just because patients believe that they are receiving effective treatment.

- *Hawthorne effect* – the Hawthorne effect is the finding that for every change in circumstances there will be a change in behaviour.

- *Attentional effects* – in attentional effects, subjects may react favourably to a treatment just because they are the centre of a lot of attention.

- *Motivational effects* – motivational effects are the result of a subject trying much harder just because they have been singled out for treatment and made to feel special.

(Dyslexia Association of Ireland 2005, reproduced with permission)

Even taking the above into account, there is no doubt in my mind that dyslexics can and do benefit from some alternative therapies – for relaxation, social interaction, personal development and self-esteem.

A word of caution

There are two main problems that people should be aware of with regard to complementary and alternative therapies. First, in the UK (as in most countries), with the exception of osteopathy and chiropractic, none of the complementary medical disciplines are as yet state registered. This means that anyone can set up as a practitioner and they do not, in the eyes of the law, need to be qualified. It is therefore worthwhile to approach established practitioners with a track record, or talking to others who have been treated at the same practice.

Second, as mentioned above, many of these therapies have not been evaluated in scientific studies. There is often little or no evidence about the safety or effectiveness of a therapy. Unlike conventional medicine which has to go through years of testing to prove its safety, there is no such requirement for alternative therapies. Therapists claim that because the therapies have been used for thousands of years – they must be safe. Many doctors are calling for complementary and alternative therapies to be regulated in the same way as traditional medicine. The problem is it is extremely difficult to carry out clinical trials and prove not only their effectiveness, but more importantly their safety, because many of the characteristics of these treatments make it difficult or impossible to conduct proper clinical trials.

Most practitioners belong to their own professional organizations, which regulate and monitor their actions. These organizations, in turn, can register with professional bodies (see Useful addresses) such as:

- British Complementary Medical Association (BCMA)
- Complementary Medical Association (CMA)
- Institute for Complementary Medicine (ICM)
- National Centre for Complementary and Alternative Medicine (NCCAM).

Take care when looking for a therapist

In theory, anyone can set themselves up as a 'therapist' and charge fees with very little, if any, experience. You only have to log onto the internet or read a newspaper to find lots of so called 'universities' advertising degrees given in almost anything in exchange for a fee. The problem is that these certificates can look very real!

Some therapies are regulated by their own professional body and it is always a good idea to check out whether the therapist you are looking to use belongs to such an organization and whether they are registered. These organizations usually offer some type of insurance cover for their members.

Do your homework

Word of mouth is the best recommendation. However, if the therapy is very specialized or new you may not be able to find anyone who has used it before. You may then find the following guidelines helpful:

1. Is the therapist qualified?

2. What qualifications does the therapist have?

3.   Where was he trained?

4.   Is he registered with a professional body?

5.   Does the therapist have a certificate and can you see it?

6.   How long has this type of therapy been in use?

7.   Does the therapist have ongoing training?

8.   What experience does the therapist have?

9.   Can they give you names and telephone numbers of similar people they have treated?

10.   Does the therapist claim to 'cure' dyslexia?

11.   Is there any research to support claims that the therapy works?

12.   Consider whether it could be dangerous – e.g. flashing lights can sometimes cause epilepsy.

13.   How much does the treatment cost?

14.   Will you get your money back if it does not work?

Chapter 2

IDENTIFYING LEARNING DIFFICULTIES

Many parents feel overwhelmed and often do not know where to turn when their child has dyslexia or specific learning difficulties (SpLDs). Dyslexia may not carry the stigma of years ago, but you are still left with the feeling that your child is the odd one out and what on earth you are going to do about it.

Because I have written this book, does not mean that I do not believe in traditional teaching methods – on the contrary. I believe we should first identify if there actually is a problem. If you do not know exactly what is wrong, how can you put the correct help and support in place? When you know the exact nature of the problems then you can go about trying to alleviate them.

There have been many research papers to support the fact that children with dyslexia should be taught using multisensory teaching methods – especially phonics (National Research Council 1998; National Reading Panel undated; Lyon undated). Indeed, the majority of children respond well to phonic-based teaching, not just children with learning difficulties. Once you have a sound basic teaching programme in place, then it might be appropriate to look at whether alternative therapies could also help. I cannot stress enough that without the basis of good teaching methods, it is highly unlikely that alternative therapies could work.

Therapists working in the developmental delay, visual and massage areas might say that children need only to use their particular therapy for the child to be 'cured'. They may well say that their 'products' can work on their own. However, in my experience and in the best interest of the child, it is advisable to use the following steps:

1. Test to find out if the child has a problem.

2. Put a multisensory education plan in place.

3.   Look at the alternative therapies available.

Dyslexia and specific learning difficulties

Dyslexia and specific learning difficulties (SpLDs) often come under the same umbrella, causing confusion, especially among parents. Dyslexia/specific learning difficulties affect 4% of the population. Problems can reveal themselves in reading, writing, number work, short-term memory, hand control and visual processing. Timekeeping, sense of direction and interpersonal skills can also be affected. These difficulties often result in great frustration, particularly bearing in mind that diagnosed dyslexics are often of high or above average intelligence.

Approximately 75% to 80% of people with dyslexia are male. Many dyslexic people are extremely bright in lots of ways, always talking and asking questions, yet they do not seem to reach their full potential in the academic field. Early identification is key because once you identify that a child has a learning difficulty and rule out any medical problems, you can start to work towards a solution. Without identification it is difficult to put in the necessary help or support. Many people with dyslexia also have other specific learning difficulties, most commonly dyscalculia, dysgraphia, dyspraxia or attention deficit hyperactivity disorder, so I have included information about all of these learning difficulties below.

Dyslexia in children
Early identification checklist

The signs below may indicate that a pre-school child is dyslexic – they do not need to have all of these problems. However, if these problems continue beyond the time that the average child has grown out of them, they may indicate dyslexia and advice should be sought. For a more detailed introduction to dyslexia, you may also want to read *An Introduction to Dyslexia for Parents and Professionals* (Hultquist 2006).

WEAKNESSES

1.   Is there a family history of learning difficulties?

2.   Did the child have delayed speech, a lisp or is the speech unclear?

3.   Does he have problems getting dressed, putting shoes on the correct feet, doing up buttons, laces, etc.?

4.   Does he enjoy hearing stories but shows no interest in the written word?

5. Do people continually say he is lazy and not paying attention?

6. Does he have problems with games:

    - tripping

    - bumping

    - falling over

    - catching a ball

    - skipping

    - hopping?

7. Can he clap a rhythm back?

8. Does he often accidentally say blue is green, red is yellow, etc.?

9. Does he often have to search for words and often mislabel them?

10. Does he confuse under/over, up/down?

11. Can he select the odd word out, i.e. cat, mat, pig, fat?

12. Can he put things in sequence:

    - nursery rhymes

    - numbers up to ten

    - days of the week

    - alphabet

    - using coloured beads, thread green, red, blue, white correctly?

13. Does he grip pencils and pens too tightly?

STRENGTHS

1. Is he quick thinking and does he have a lot of original thought?

2. Is he good at creativity, art/colour?

3. Does he have an aptitude for construction games like building blocks, or remote control and keyboards?

4. Does he appear bright but unable to do simple things?

Children's checklist

The signs below may indicate a child is dyslexic. They do not need to have all of these problems. However, if these problems continue beyond the time that the average child has grown out of them, they may indicate dyslexia and advice should be sought.

READING AND SPELLING

When your child reads and spells, does he frequently:

- confuse letters that look similar: d – b, u – n, m – n?
- confuse letters that sound the same: v, f, th?
- reverse words: was – saw, now – won?
- transpose words: left – felt?
- read a word correctly and then further down the page read it wrongly?
- change the words around: the cat sat on the mat (the mat sat on the cat)?
- confuse small words: of, for, from?
- have difficulty when reading in keeping the correct place on a line and frequently loses his place?
- read correctly but does not understand what he is reading?

WRITING

Even after frequent instruction does he still:

- not know whether to use his right or left hand?
- leave out capital letters or use them in the wrong places?
- forget to dot 'i' and cross 't'?
- form letters and numbers badly?
- use margins and does his writing slope on the page?
- use punctuation and paragraphs in the wrong places or not at all?

OTHER INDICATIONS

1. Is there a family history of dyslexia or similar difficulties?

2. Was he a late developer?

3. Is he easily distracted and has poor concentration?

4. Does he get confused between left/right, east/west, up/down, over/under?

5. Does he have sequencing difficulties:

    - alphabet

    - nursery rhymes

    - months of the year

    - numbers in tables?

6. Does he hold a pen too tightly and awkwardly?

7. Does he have problems telling the time?

8. Does he have problems with tying shoe laces, etc.?

9. Does he have short-term memory problems related to printed words and instructions?

10. Does he have mixed laterality (i.e. uses either right or left hands or eyes in writing and other tasks)?

11. Does he have particular difficulty copying from a blackboard?

12. Does he have confusion with mathematical symbols (plus/minus etc.)?

13. Does he have an inability to follow more than one instruction at a time?

14. Is he unable to use a dictionary or telephone directory?

Adult dyslexia

Dyslexic people are often highly creative and original. They usually succeed through sheer hard work and determination. They are valuable members of a working team. Many dyslexics excel in areas such as:

- architecture

- arts

- computer sciences

- construction

- electronics

- engineering
- entertainment
- mathematics
- physics
- sports.

Many adults who have dyslexia have never been diagnosed as such. It is only now that some of them are coming to realize that they have a recognized problem and are seeking help. Dyslexics often have major difficulties in a work environment; performing tasks such as filling in forms and try to hide their problems. Many adult dyslexics suffer from low self-esteem, lack of confidence and fall short of their employment ability. They are often relieved to know that their lack of progress is due to dyslexia and, once diagnosed, they can receive the right kind of help.

Checklist

Some of the problems listed below may indicate that an adult has dyslexia but the person does not need to have all of these problems. Do you:

- have a family history of dyslexia?
- remember having problems when you were at school?
- have problems with reading?
- take a long time to read?
- have to re-read the same piece several times?
- keep losing your place?
- miss off endings of words?
- miss words out?
- read correctly but not understand what you are reading?

When writing, do you:

- find it difficult to take notes?
- produce 'messy' work?
- not know where to start?
- have poor punctuation?
- make lots of mistakes when spelling?

- have good days and bad days with spelling?
- miss off endings of words?
- reverse letters or leave them out?
- have difficulty filling in forms, timesheets, etc.?
- have problems using a dictionary or telephone directory?
- have problems recalling the months of the year forwards and backwards?

Do you have problems:

- reading maps and directions?
- with left/right?
- with telling the time?
- with time management, getting to appointments on time?

With numbers do you:

- have difficulties with mental arithmetic?
- reverse numbers or leave them out?
- have problems repeating numbers backwards, i.e. 863, 368?
- mix up numbers, i.e. 13 and 31?
- often dial the wrong telephone number?
- have problems doing sums in your head?

Dyscalculia

Dyscalculia is a specific learning difficulty relating to mathematics. Like dyslexia, dyscalculia can be caused by a visual perceptual deficit. Dyscalculia refers specifically to the inability to perform operations in maths or arithmetic. It could be described as an extreme difficulty with numbers. Just as there is no single set of signs that characterize all dyslexics, there is no one cause of dyscalculia.

We still do not know very much about this condition, but it is thought that around 3% of the UK population may have it. Around 60% of dyslexics have difficulties with dyscalculia and yet it was only in 2003 that a test for screening for dyscalculia was developed (Butterworth 2003). It is hoped that over the next few years we shall begin to understand this a little more. See Butterworth 2005 for a discussion of developmental dyscalculia.

Checklist

The signs below may indicate a child is dyscalculic. They do not need to have all of these problems. However, if these problems continue beyond the time that the average child has grown out of them, they may indicate dyscalculia and advice should be sought. Does your child frequently:

- confuse numbers, i.e. 51 for 15?
- transpose and reverse numbers, when reading or writing?
- confuse: minus, subtract, take away?
- confuse: add, plus, add on?

Does he have problems:

- learning the times tables?
- working out simple money and change?
- estimating numbers: tens, hundreds, thousands?
- working out percentages?
- working out averages?
- understanding $2 + 5 = 7$ (but does not have problems with $5 + 2 = 7$)?
- working out the speed miles per hour?
- telling the time?
- learning the date?
- answering questions correctly but being unable to tell you how he got the answer?

Dyscalculia may not have the same stigma surrounding it, but it is very important that it is recognized as soon as possible. If these problems are not picked up at an early age, they impact on a child's self-esteem and it all takes a long time to correct.

Dysgraphia

Dysgraphia is the inability to write properly, despite a student being given adequate time and attention. The cause of this disorder is still unknown but is thought it could be due to a language disorder and/or damage to the motor system. There is ongoing research to try to establish exactly what causes it and how people can be helped.

If people are suffering with dysgraphia, the main sign is that their handwriting will be barely legible. The writing will appear incorrect or distorted and have letters of different sizes and spaces. This could be a ploy because if someone cannot read your writing they cannot tell if it is spelt properly. Some people with dyslexic-type problems may therefore deliberately write scruffily, so people cannot tell if it is spelt wrong. However, it is usually a problem with the actual physical side of writing.

Checklist

The signs below may indicate that someone has dysgraphia. They do not need to have all of these problems. However, if these problems continue beyond the time that the average person has grown out of them, they may indicate dysgraphia and advice should be sought.

1. Written text very poor considering language development.

2. Poor motor control.

3. Writing that is almost impossible to read.

4. Mixture of printing and cursive writing on the same line.

5. Writes in all directions, i.e. right slant then left slant.

6. Big and small spaces between words.

7. Different-sized letters on the same line.

8. Mixes up capital letters and lower case letters on the same line.

9. Abnormal and irregular formation of letters.

10. Very slow writing.

11. Very slow copying from board.

12. Does not follow margins.

13. Grips the pen too tightly and with a 'fist grip'.

14. Holds pen very low down so fingers almost touch the paper.

15. Watches hand intently whilst actually writing.

16. Poor spelling.

17.   Bizarre spelling.

18.   Problems with spelling wrong words, i.e. 'brot' for brought and 'stayshun' for station.

19.   Problems with spelling words such as drink as 'brink'.

Dyspraxia

Dyspraxia is also called developmental dyspraxia or developmental coordination disorder (DCD). It is not certain what causes dyspraxia but it is thought to be due to an immaturity in neurone development in the brain. Dyspraxia affects approximately 10% of the population, some severely. The overwhelming majority are male.

Some people may be only affected slightly, others more seriously. Sometimes developmental milestones are delayed and there might be speech difficulties. Not surprisingly, this leads on to difficulties at school. Often dyspraxia is accompanied by difficulties in vision and movement, i.e. problems with catching a ball.

Checklist

Following is a checklist on dyspraxia. However, you must remember that when children start school they may make several of the mistakes listed. It is only if these symptoms continue beyond the time that the average child has grown out of them that they may indicate dyspraxia and advice should be sought. Children who fall over, drop things and generally take longer to do things are not necessarily suffering with dyspraxia.

INFANTS

Very young children may have delayed milestones, including problems with:

- sleeping
- being fretful and fidgeting
- sitting up (keep falling over)
- 'bum shuffling' rather than crawling
- walking late
- talking late and speech problems
- messy eating

- baby puzzles or building blocks
- picking up small items.

CHILDREN

Older children may have the same problems as infants, including:

- fidgeting constantly
- never sitting still
- when sitting, swinging his legs and fiddling with his hands and anything else around him
- knocking things over
- spilling everything
- problems using knives and forks
- bumping into everything all the time
- stumbling into doors
- falling over for no apparent reason
- problems using stairs and steps
- difficulties standing on tiptoe or one leg
- problems dressing and doing up buttons
- trouble doing up shoelaces
- problems telling the time.

When playing the child may have problems with:

- fine motor skills
- puzzles, construction games, building blocks, etc.
- using scissors and craft tools
- painting and colouring small areas
- threading a needle
- catching or kicking a ball
- hitting a moving ball, i.e. tennis, etc.
- riding a bike

- using roller skates
- coordination for swimming.

In a more formal setting such as a classroom, teachers may notice that the child has the following problems:

- When reading has difficulty in keeping the correct place on a line and frequently loses his place.
- When writing, grips the pencil very tightly and awkwardly.
- When writing, changes hands constantly and does not know whether to use his right or left hand.
- Writes in different directions on the same paper.
- Does not use margins.
- Writing slopes on page.
- Copying symbols, i.e. circles, squares, and triangles.
- Copying work from whiteboards, etc.
- Following instructions.
- Reading maps.

Whilst there is still no known treatment for dyspraxia, it is generally thought that physiotherapy and occupational therapy can help to improve motor and coordination skills. There are lots of things you can do at home to help, with balancing games, trampettes, wobble boards, standing on one leg, etc. What makes these particularly helpful is that fact that they are fun.

Attention deficit hyperactivity disorder

Attention deficit hyperactivity disorder (ADHD) has been known about for a long time. It has undergone several name changes, one time being known as hyperkinesias (Latin derivative for 'super active'), hyperactivity, ADD and latterly ADHD (with or without hyperactivity). As with other problems mentioned in this book, there are different degrees of severity. A large proportion of children with ADHD display features of dyslexia and dyspraxia.

A child who cannot concentrate, who moves around constantly, has poor school performance (in contrast with his intelligence) and displays disruptive behaviour may be suffering with ADHD. There is evidence to suggest that children with this problem could eventually be expelled from school and/or be in trouble with the police. You do not grow out of ADHD, but you do learn to modify your behaviour.

At times all children may have periods of being overactive and inattentive, but hyperactive children are disruptive nearly all the time. ADHD is thought to affect between 3% and 5% of the school-age population, although it is difficult to establish the exact percentage.

Checklist

The signs below may indicate a person has ADHD. They do not need to have all of these problems. However, if these problems continue beyond the time that their peers have grown out of them, they may indicate ADHD and advice should be sought.

INFANTS

Very young children may often appear distressed in the following ways:

- extreme restlessness
- poor sleep patterns
- difficult to feed
- excessive thirst
- constant thirst
- dry skin
- frequent tantrums
  - screaming
  - head banging
  - rocking the cot.

CHILDREN

Older children may become fearless and impulsive and display the following characteristics:

- not stopping to think
- taking undue risks
- dashing around
- erratic behaviour

- prone to accidents
- increased activity – always on the go
- compulsive touching everything and everyone
- clumsiness
- talking incessantly
- allergies
- sleep and appetite problems.

The child may have poor coordination and experience the following problems:

- tying laces
- dressing
- handwriting
- ball games
- lack self-esteem
- making friends
- impatience, so won't take turns in games
- demands must be met immediately
- may hit out and grab things.

The child may also show signs of an inflexible personality by being:

- uncooperative
- defiant
- disobedient.

In a more formal setting such as a classroom, teachers may also notice problems with:

- poor concentration and brief attention span
- sitting through lessons
- constant fidgeting
- constant moving of feet, hands, etc.
- tapping pens, pencils, books, etc.
- roaming around the classroom

- taking turns

- blurting out answers to questions

- speaking entirely inappropriately out of turn

- weak short-term memory

- normal or high IQ but underperformance at school.

ADULTS

Adults with ADHD present with the following problems:

- Most of the features of ADHD in childhood remain.

- Employment may be difficult because of relationship problems and poor memory.

- Antisocial behaviour may become so extreme that it leads to trouble with the law and excess alcohol consumption.

- Poor self-esteem may be distressing.

In the past, ADHD has been perceived as the fault of the parents – that the children are merely naughty and their parents need to be stricter with them. It has been over 20 years since a link with fatty acid deficiency was found and it would be of great benefit to these children if a routine test was available to them.

Summing up

The term specific learning difficulty covers a wide range of problems: the biggest being to identify exactly what is wrong. Without this, it is difficult to put in the correct and necessary help to support the child. Most children with SpLDs stay in mainstream schooling with some additional help; hardly any children need to attend special schools. For useful addresses, please go to p.122.

Chapter 3

HEARING

With so much research carried out over the last few decades, it is now universally accepted that some dyslexics have problems with auditory skills (Schulte-Körne, Deimel, Bartling *et al.* 1998). Some people who go for a standard hearing test can be given the 'all clear' and yet still be suffering from a form of hearing problem. This seems to be because some people appear to be hypersensitive to certain sounds/frequencies or have asymmetrical hearing. If someone perceives sounds differently in their right to their left ear, this can lead to problems with sound discrimination – a major problem for dyslexics.

Another consideration when looking at auditory problems is the crucial part that the brain plays. Most of the therapies described in this chapter are designed to normalize the auditory system, thereby changing how the brain processes and organizes the input received from the ears. Most of them look at the possibility of 'normalizing' hearing to aid learning. If you choose to have any of these treatments, a full assessment of the person's auditory system should be conducted to ascertain if they are suitable for the type of therapy on offer. The therapies described include:

- Tomatis
- Auditory Integration Training (AIT)
- Lexiphone
- Interactive Metronome®
- Spectral Activated Music of Optimal Natural Structure (SAMONAS)
- music therapy

I have included a short auditory checklist below which includes some suggestions to help identify whether the child actually has a hearing problem.

Listening checklist

This checklist is a tool to see if you or your child may have a listening problem. We cannot 'see' listening. The only way to 'get at it' is indirectly through skills that are related to it in one way or another. This checklist, developed by Canadian Tomatis practitioner Paul Madaule, is from *When Listening Comes Alive* (Madaule 1993). It offers a catalogue of abilities, skills or qualities that will enable you to assess whether you or your child may have a listening problem. There is no score. This is simply a tool for you to evaluate your own or your child's ability to listen, and thus to learn. Check as many boxes as you feel appropriate.

Listening checklist

Developmental history
Our early years

This knowledge about our younger years is extremely important in early identification and prevention of listening problems. It also sheds light on possible causes of listening problems.

☐ A stressful pregnancy	☐ Delay in motor development
☐ Difficult birth	☐ Delay in language development
☐ Adoption	☐ Recurring ear infections
☐ Early separation from mother	

Receptive listening
Our external environment

This type of listening is directed outward to the world around us. It keeps us attuned to what's going on at home, at work, in the classroom or with friends.

☐ Short attention span	☐ Confusion of similar sounding words
☐ Distractibility	☐ Frequent need for repetition
☐ Oversensitivity to sounds	☐ Inability to follow sequential instructions
☐ Misinterpretation of questions	

Expressive listening
Our internal atmosphere

This is the kind of listening that is directed within us. We use it to listen to ourselves and to gauge and control our voice when we speak and sing.

☐ Flat and monotonous voice	☐ Inability to sing in tune
☐ Hesitant speech	☐ Confusion or reversal of letters
☐ Weak vocabulary	☐ Poor reading comprehension
☐ Poor sentence structure	☐ Poor reading aloud
☐ Overuse of stereotyped expressions	☐ Poor spelling

Motor skills
Our physical abilities

The ear of the body (the vestibule), which controls balance, muscle and eye coordination and body image, needs close scrutiny also.

☐ Poor posture	☐ Hard time with organization, structure
☐ Fidgety behavior	☐ Confusion of left and right
☐ Clumsy, uncoordinated movements	☐ Mixed dominance (of hands?)
☐ Poor sense of rhythm	☐ Poor sports skills
☐ Messy handwriting	

The level of energy
Our fuel system

The ear acts like a dynamo (a powerful motor), providing us with the "brain" energy we need not only to survive but also to lead fulfilling lives.

☐ Difficulty getting up	☐ Hyperactivity
☐ Tiredness at the end of the day	☐ Tendency toward depression
☐ Habit of procrastinating	☐ Feeling overburdened with everyday tasks

Behavioral and social adjustment
Our relationship skills

A listening difficulty is often related to these qualities of interacting with others.

☐ Low tolerance for frustration	☐ Tendency to withdraw or to avoid others
☐ Poor self-confidence	☐ Irritability
☐ Poor self-image	☐ Immaturity
☐ Shyness	☐ Low motivation, no interest in school/work
☐ Difficulty making friends	☐ Negative attitude toward school/work

Source: Madaule, P. (1993) *When Listening Comes Alive*. Norval, Ontario: Moulin, pp.191–2. Reproduced with permission.

Tomatis

In 1982 Dr Alfred Tomatis, a French ear, nose and throat specialist, invented a device called the Electronic Ear. Tomatis used this device to normalize hearing and the way the brain processes information. He believed that the root cause of many learning difficulties was due to the way we listen and if we did not listen 'properly' we could have impaired hearing, which in turn could lead to dyslexia. He went on to develop a highly effective technique to remedy this problem. It is said that Tomatis' groundbreaking work led to a new multidisciplinary science called Audio-Psycho-Phonology (APP).

Tomatis was highly respected in the medical field. He was named Knight of Public Health of France in 1951 and later received the gold medal for scientific research. He wrote numerous books and articles. There are now over 200 Tomatis centres worldwide. Tomatis was not only known in his field, but also one of the first audiologists who believed that dyslexia was related more to the ear than the eye (as is the belief in other medical areas).

How does it work?

Tomatis used a device called the Electronic Ear to deliver treatments, which works by simulating the stages of listening development. Special headphones equipped with a bone-conduction sensor deliver sound through a sophisticated stereo system. The sensor captures vibrations through the bone. Lower frequencies are filtered out so that only the 'proper' sounds are heard.

The method uses specially modified auditory feedback in a broad range of frequencies. This approach is extremely useful for children with auditory processing problems. A lot of people with dyslexia have auditory processing problems. The patients using the Tomatis method spend a number of hours each day listening through headphones to Mozart and similar music (sometimes, if appropriate, they listen to their mother's voice). There are various filters which can be applied and adjusted through the device. These treatments aim to re-pattern a child's hearing range.

How many sessions are needed?

Patients using the Tomatis method have an average of 70 hours therapy, usually split into half-hour sessions.

Who will benefit most?

Tomatis worked for over 40 years and it is claimed that in that time he successfully treated children with auditory processing problems, dyslexia and other learning difficulties.

Auditory Integration Training

Auditory Integration Training (AIT) was developed in 1982 by Dr Guy Bérard, a French ear, nose and throat specialist, to normalize hearing and the way the brain processes information. Bérard realized that many people with acute hearing problems often had learning disorders such as dyslexia, ADHD and other learning difficulties. AIT works on a sensory-based treatment and has its base in the Tomatis method. Its aim is to retrain the auditory system.

How does it work?

Bérard invented a device called an audiokinetron to exercise the ear. The audiokinetron randomizes and filters the frequencies from music and sends these sounds into the patient's ears through headphones. This enables a person's perception of hearing to be retrained.

Some people have different hearing levels in each ear. Others can have hearing problems which include hypersensitivity to certain frequencies. When right and left ears perceive sounds in different ways this can lead to poor sound discrimination, resulting in learning difficulties.

How many sessions are needed?

Patients listen to this gentle music for ten hours, usually split into half-hour sessions.

Who will benefit most?

AIT helps people with dyslexia and other learning difficulties by developing better concentration and awareness of decreased sound sensitivity. Some students with ADHD have also reported less impulsivity and restlessness and reduction in distractibility. Bérard's book *Hearing Equals Behaviour* (2000) has some good case samples.

Lexiphone

The Lexiphone method was developed in the mid-1970s by a psychiatrist and professor of psychology, Dr Isi Beller, who has spent more than 25 years researching dyslexia.

How does it work?

An audio-feedback uses artificial means to re-educate automatic language processing without the awareness of the student. The client's voice can be played back through headphones equipped with a built-in microphone creating an auditory feedback loop.

The Lexiphone method retrains auditory attention and speech awareness during selected listening, speaking, reading and writing activities.

The training is split into three phases. The first phase, or re-education, engages students in nonlinguistic entertaining activities such as puzzles, drawing, etc. whilst listening to music or speech. During this phase the client is restructuring the elements that make up his language without even being aware of it. The second and third phases each build on the previous work.

Who can use the Lexiphone method?

Lexiphone classes are taught by a speech-language therapist who is specially trained in the Lexiphone method.

How many sessions are needed?

Clients usually require between 90 and 150 45-minute sessions.

Who will benefit most?

The Lexiphone method is said to help people with auditory problems and dyslexia.

Interactive Metronome®

For centuries musicians have used a metronome to help them keep time. It has been used in the last few years with people suffering from Parkinson's disease and stroke patients. However, more recently the method has created attention as more work is being carried out with clients with dyslexia and ADHD. An experimental study of 56 boys, 9 to 12 years old, diagnosed with ADHD found those undergoing IM treatment (19 subjects) showed significant improvements compared to a control group (18 subjects) and a video–placebo group (19 subjects) (Schaffer *et al.* 2001).

Interactive Metronome® (IM) therapy is claimed, amongst other things, to effect improvement in attention and concentration, motor control and coordination.

How does it work?

Quite simply, a metronome works by keeping time. Clients with dyslexia and ADHD have difficulty processing different sounds and staying on task. Interactive Metronome® therapists use metronomes to help the client focus, pay attention to certain sounds and block out all other noises. The metronome helps train the brain to plan, sequence and process information more effectively through repetition of interactive exercises. The Interactive Metronome® programme involves repeated hand, toe and heel exercises. These exercises can be varied and extended so that clients are able to perform thousands of repetitions, which are carried out while auditory guide tones direct the individual to keep in time with the metronome beat.

Who can use IM?

Metronome therapy is being successfully used by occupational therapists, physical therapists and speech therapists.

How many sessions are needed?

The treatment consists of one-hour sessions and can be completed in three to five weeks.

Who will benefit most?

Interactive Metronome® therapy is said to help people with many disorders, including Asperger's syndrome, autism, ADHD and dyslexia.

SAMONAS

SAMONAS is an acronym of Spectral Activated Music of Optimal Natural Structure. It is another form of electronically tailored music therapy, developed in Germany by the physicist Ingo Steinbach.

How does it work?

The system is said to train the auditory system to process the full range of sound without distortion, hypersensitivity or frequency loss.

Who will benefit most?

SAMONAS is said to help people with hearing loss, impaired speech, hypersensitive hearing, auditory processing problems, ADHD, dyslexia and other difficulties. Some therapists claim it can also help with auditory discrimination problems. A lot of people with dyslexia have auditory discrimination problems.

Can this be done at home?

The UK National Academy for Child Development can supply an individualized treatment plan for use at home. Clients listen to SAMONAS discs five days a week, for variable time scales. The CDs contain classical music and nature sounds that have been specially adapted.

Music therapy

We are all aware that a rousing piece of music can lift our spirits, whether it is a soft ballad to relax and help us unwind or heavy metal music which can send some of us into frenzy. When you visit a doctor's surgery they often have soft music playing in the background. Supermarkets use music (muzak) to promote shopping: if they are very busy they will play something in quick time and noisy; when they are quiet they may change to soft muzak, encouraging us to spend more time and money.

Music therapy is used within a therapeutic relationship to address physical, emotional, cognitive and social needs.

How does it work?

Music therapy is practised by therapists who use their training as musicians, clinicians and researchers to effect changes in cognitive, physical and emotional skills. The music therapist assesses the strengths and needs of each client and then indicates the type of treatment required. This could involve singing, creating, dancing to and listening to music. Usually patient and therapist take an active part in music therapy by playing and singing together. The therapist does not teach, but encourages the use of instruments and the patient's own voice to explore the world of sound.

There are different approaches to music therapy, just as there are in all other therapies. A lot depends on the needs of the client. A wide variety of styles is needed in order to complement the individual needs of each client. Through therapy the therapist aims to facilitate positive changes in emotional state and well-being. Music therapy helps people by developing better concentration and awareness of decreased sound sensitivity.

It is said that music therapy can reduce heart rate, blood pressure, pain and anxiety. It is used in hospitals to alleviate pain, improve patients' moods and counteract depression. It has even been used for women in labour. It can promote calm and induce sleep.

How many sessions are needed?

This varies from client to client, but would usually be for approximately ten hours, usually split into half-hour sessions.

Who will benefit most?

Music therapy can be used to help people with dyslexia, ADHD and other learning difficulties by helping with auditory discrimination of sounds (a major problem for dyslexic people) and with organizational skills. It also encourages clients to stay calm and increases creativity. Clients who have used this therapy say they have an improved attention span, better memory skills and increased self-esteem.

Music therapy has been shown to be beneficial for people with dyslexia, ADHD and other learning difficulties. Clients develop a greater sense of awareness and confidence, which in turn leads to improved self-esteem. Music therapists work in a variety of locations including hospitals, day centres, prisons and schools.

Qualifications

Most music therapists have undergraduate and/or graduate degrees in music therapy and must keep their qualifications up to date.

Summing up

As you can see, there are many treatments available for evaluating auditory problems. Sometimes all that is required is a quick and simple hearing test. Others require more in-depth testing and training. Auditory training may sound quite complicated but it simply means fully testing the ears and training them to listen and respond to appropriate treatment. This treatment may take a few months or several years. If successful it can be a tremendous help to the client. However, to add a word of caution, just as with the other alternative/complementary therapies in this book, some of these therapies can be very expensive and go on for a long time. For useful addresses, please go to p.122.

Chapter 4

BODYWORKS

Many of the therapies listed in this chapter are well known and require little expla-
nation. All the 'bodyworks' therapies work in a holistic and natural way to promote
good health by manipulating the body (or parts of it), which in turn strengthens
the immune system, helps to flush out toxins and provides stimulation and relaxation. Many of these therapists work alongside medical professionals and doctors
may refer clients to them. There are a significant number of therapies that work in
similar ways, including:

- Chiropractic
- Physiotherapy and occupational therapy
- Osteopathy
- Alexander technique
- Yoga
- Pilates
- Feldenkrais
- Zero Balancing.

Chiropractic by Christopher Vickers

Chiropractic is defined as the science and art of detecting and correcting dysfunctional areas (known in the jargon as subluxations) of the pelvis, spine and skull
(cranium) that cause interference in the normal functioning of the nervous system
which these structures either house, support or protect.

As the nervous system is the organizer and regulator of all bodily functions, it
has become well known within the profession, and by patients who have received

treatment from chiropractors, that correction of these dysfunctional areas can have far-reaching positive effects on many areas of the body. It is because of this interconnectedness that both practitioners and patients have reported beneficial effects with regard to dyslexia/dyspraxia type problems, purely as a spin-off from correction of other areas relating to a particular symptom that a person has presented with.

Chiropractic originated in the USA in 1895 when a magnetic healer, D.D. Palmer, corrected a misaligned vertebra in the spine of a local janitor. This had the effect of curing the deafness the man had experienced in one ear for the previous 17 years. Despite opposition from medical authorities, the profession has developed into being the third largest primary healthcare provider in the western world after medicine and dentistry.

At a similar time, also in the United States, osteopathy was developing along similar lines, although they believed that spinal and pelvic dysfunction disturbed blood flow rather than nerve function. In the early part of the 1900s an engineer, M.B. De Jarnette, was injured in a factory explosion and sought treatment from the founder of osteopathy, Andrew Taylor Still. De Jarnette was encouraged by Still to become an osteopath and he went on to become a chiropractor.

At this time cranial osteopaths were having great results with Still's techniques, but were also noticing some unexpected adverse reactions. De Jarnette discovered a method by which he could reproducibly correct pelvic dysfunction, which simultaneously minimized the frequency of adverse reactions to cranial corrections. He developed his research over many years into a well known and widely practised chiropractic technique – Sacro-Occipital Technique (SOT) – which highlighted the functional relationship of pelvis and cranium.

Many chiropractors and osteopaths have studied cranial dysfunction and correction intensively. Through clinical observation it was noticed that practitioners who specialized in cranial work were often able to help people (especially children) with learning or behavioural difficulties. At first this was difficult to quantify and predict. After careful study and organization, this work has developed significantly from De Jarnette and Still's original methods. The art and science of muscle testing, Applied Kinesiology (AK), was developed by an American chiropractor called George Goodheart. His methods helped evaluate cranial problems and along with sacro-occipital and other chiropractic techniques have advanced the study of cranial dysfunction with regard to correcting dyslexic/dyspraxic problems.

It is now understood that proper eye function is of major significance in learning, as well as the efficient delivery of the sensory ocular (eye) information to the visual centre of the brain and the distribution of this information either into

motor function (i.e. performing and action) or sensory assimilation (i.e. comprehension, imagination or memory).

If a person has cranial (or spinal/pelvic) dysfunction then interference can
occur both directly to cranial nerves, especially the third (occulomotor) cranial nerve
which regulates eye muscle movements, as well as indirectly, to interfere with
correct assimilation and mental processing of sensory eye information. Either or
both of these scenarios can result in inappropriate eye movements (which may
reduce reading speed and effectiveness, due to alteration of normal eye scanning)
or alter the processing of information into the brain, therefore possibly interfering
with understanding and memory mechanisms. This may be due to faulty function
of the second (optic) cranial nerve or poor crossover of the information into both
sides of the brain.

Correction of faulty pelvic, spinal or cranial mechanics can alter the functioning of the membranes (sheaths) that surround the spinal cord and brain. It is
believed that incorrect balance between these membranes has both a direct and
indirect influence upon the electrical functioning of the brain. The chiropractic
sacro-occipital cranial and muscle testing (AK) techniques make the most of these
connections for both identifying and correcting problems. The corrections are
very gentle and may involve soothing light, moulding of the skull bones or placing
special blocks under the pelvis while encouraging certain breathing patterns.

Another American chiropractor, C. Ferreri, developed a system of muscle
testing various nerve circuits in the body, known as reflexes, that are concerned
with the four primal survival systems of man – feeding, fight/flight, reproduction
and the immune systems. He noted that all bodily functions must work within or
through these survival systems in an organized and integrated manner. Various
forms of stress, including physical, emotional, chemical or environmental trauma,
can and do interfere with the organized function of these reflex systems.

Ferreri's technique, Neural Organization Technique (NOT), was a synthesis of
AK and SOT. Early in its development, the organizational effect of NOT on the
nervous system was recognized as successfully influencing the treatment of
dyslexia/learning difficulties. A specific deficit in the vestibular (balance) and ocular
(visual) reflex system was found to be present in this condition. As a result many chiropractors and kinesiologists became interested in learning how to address these and
other conditions which have resisted the best efforts of orthodox treatment.

As a result of NOT work, which involves stimulating reflex areas on the body
in a specific sequence, often with the person changing eye function as directed (i.e.
eyes open/closed), it was also noted that many other conditions were helped
including the frequently identified attention deficit disorder (ADD) and attention
deficit hyperactivity disorder (ADHD) which often require more extensive

treatment protocols. These reflex stimulations are thought to clear dysfunctional nerve programmes in the spinal cord and brain. No drugs are ever used in the correction of these conditions.

Chiropractors and osteopaths who have developed an interest in this type of work have shown that various exercises are frequently helpful in assisting corrections, as well as maintaining the gains made and preventing relapse. These may be eye exercises or hand–eye coordination exercises. However, it has been found that unless these structural (pelvic/spinal/cranial) or reflex faults are corrected, the individual is most unlikely to improve by performing corrective exercises alone. Dietary advice is commonly found to be necessary such as the encouragement to take in the correct type of essential fatty acids which help improve nerve function, plenty of raw fruits and vegetables, and drinking plenty of water.

Correction of these conditions is best undertaken by a team approach with good communication between team members. The team is likely but not exclusively to include an educational psychologist, optician, nutritionist and properly qualified chiropractor/osteopath. It should go without saying that these team members should be in regular contact with the patient, parents and school teachers (if applicable) as well as with each other. They should all have a specific interest in this area of work as a prerequisite to being involved.

Physiotherapy and occupational therapy
What is physiotherapy?
Physiotherapy is a science-based approach concerned with human function and movement. It uses a physical approach to promote, maintain and restore physical, psychological and social well-being. Physical therapy is the treatment of a condition, which threatens physical development.

What is occupational therapy?
Occupational therapy is a holistic therapy. Practitioners say they work on the whole system to help you reach your full potential. There are different branches of occupational therapy, some dealing exclusively with children. It is often not until children start to have physical movement problems that we realize how their educational development can be delayed.

How do occupational and physiotherapists work?
Before physiotherapists start work with clients they take an initial assessment of specific physical functions and abilities. They then discuss strategies for develop-

ing the client's difficulties with the family (if appropriate). They can offer a wide range of therapies including Sensory Integration, Bobath Neurodevelopmental Therapy, massage, mobilization, stretching, strengthening and posture education.

They work with the children, families and other people connected with the family. Each client is set achievable functional goals and given strategies to succeed in these specific tasks. These may include dressing, eating, using scissors, developing concentration levels, balance, etc. The work is always developmentally appropriate, varied, imaginative and fun. As a client gets over current problems and his needs change, so does the therapy. It is vital that enthusiastic carers are involved at home or school for optimal long-term results.

How many sessions are needed?

Therapy usually takes place for half an hour to an hour on a regular basis.

Who will benefit most?

Physiotherapists and occupational therapists see clients with a wide range of difficulties and conditions. These include developmental coordination disorders such as dyspraxia, dyslexia and other learning difficulties, back problems, postural problem and stress. People with dyslexia and other learning difficulties are known to be prone to high levels of stress. Physiotherapists and occupational therapists work in a wide range of settings, including hospitals, schools, colleges, nurseries and private homes, to achieve maximum benefits for all their clients.

Can this be done at home?

Physiotherapists and occupational therapists work with the family, school and other interested professionals and a programme is devised to be used on a regular basis.

Osteopathy

Osteopathy is a holistic therapy. Therapists say it has an effect on the whole system and they treat most conditions. It is often used with other therapies such as acupuncture and acupressure. There are different branches of osteopathy such as visceral (working on the abdominal tissues) and cranial (influencing the tone of the brain and nervous system). The aims of osteopathy are to diagnose and treat medical problems in the framework of the body. These problems could have been caused by injury or stress.

How does it work?

Osteopaths use manual techniques to help restore normal movement to joints and normal tension and elasticity to muscles and other soft tissues. Use of the hands for massaging and manipulating the framework of the body helps to remove restrictions in the muscles, nerves and blood vessels so that the patient's body is able to heal itself more effectively. Osteopathy is now seen as a mainstream complementary medicine and more and more patients are referred by doctors.

Who will benefit most?

Osteopathy can help a wide range of conditions including spinal problems, back pain and neck pain. Practitioners also treat patients with sports injuries to the muscle groups or joints of the hips, knees, ankles, feet, etc.

How many sessions are needed?

As with any treatment, time varies according to what is required. Some people return for sessions of osteopathy to keep their bodies 'in tune' while others find it is not necessary.

Alexander technique

The Alexander technique was developed by an Australian Shakespearian actor, Frederick Matthias Alexander. He had a problem with his voice and could not understand why it often seized up when he went on stage. After observing himself in a mirror, he realized he made a repeated 'unconscious movement'. The mere thought of using his voice caused him to pull his head back and tense his throat, both doing little for his performance. After scrutinizing his own and other people's movements, he noticed that others were having similar physical problems, which he attributed to incorrect posture when sitting, standing and moving and bad habits. Alexander discovered that you could rebalance the body through awareness.

Alexander eventually cured himself. He set up a practice to educate clients in the proper use of their bodies and so pioneered a method that stops people from unconsciously misusing their bodies. There are currently over 25,000 people trained in the Alexander technique throughout the world.

How does it work?

Alexander discovered that learning to use one's back well is of primary importance. He found that all body skills like speaking, playing sports and the performance of the respiratory and digestive systems are influenced by how well (or badly) your back performs. Alexander therapists believe that movement difficulties are caused by unconscious habits which interfere with poise and the capacity to learn.

By practising different movements people are made aware of how their body moves, and so relearn the posture they had when they were young. Therapists try to break the habits people have learned and teach them new ones. This leads to better breathing, improved coordination and balance and increased energy, leaving the client in a more relaxed state.

Alexander technique is taught in music and drama colleges worldwide, due to its positive influence on coordination. Out of the many alternative/complementary therapies available, the effectiveness of the Alexander technique is probably the most well documented (Barlow 2001; Garlick 1990).

How many sessions are needed?

Lessons are usually for one hour on a one-to-one basis twice a week for a three-month period. They are sometimes arranged in groups.

Who will benefit most?

The Alexander technique can be taught to anyone over six years of age and is used to relieve the symptoms of many conditions, including anxiety, asthma, back problems, postural problems and stress. People with dyslexia and other specific learning difficulties are particularly prone to stress, which produces tension (Morgan and Klein 2000; Newby, Aldridge, Sasse *et al.* 1995). Dancers, musicians and athletes, including golfers may also find it helpful.

Can this be done at home?

The Alexander technique can be carried out at home once people know how to perform the exercises. There are various DVDs and videos available (see Resourccs).

Yoga

Watch any group of young children playing – rolling around, twisting, balancing, working every muscle in the body and loving it – and you can see yoga in its most simplistic form. Yoga dates back more than 5000 years and is said to be one of the most complex exercise systems. It is a holistic spiritual discipline with its roots in eastern forms of meditation and is based on the idea of moving energy through the body: the more freely the energy flows, the healthier you feel. Yoga is said to condition the mind through physical and spiritual means, thereby keeping the body supple through movement and stretching and helping the mind through concentration and relaxation.

How does it work?

Yoga is based on a system of exercises and breathing. Pranayama is the science of proper breathing. Yoga is said to consciously work on concentrating your mind on your breathing. The average person uses approximately one-seventh of his total lung capacity. By learning how to increase this with deep breathing, you can increase the energy to various organs in the body and overcome many physical ailments.

Exercises or different postures, Asanas, are held for an extended period of time whilst breathing calmly and deeply. The Asanas are said to promote stretching, strengthening and balancing, whilst the deep breathing helps promote relaxation and mental awareness. One of the first things people may notice when they attend a yoga class is the unusual names for these exercises such as Staff Pose, Sitting Tall, The Butterfly, The Camel.

Yoga should always be carried out in a room which is relaxing, clean and quiet (and sometimes with very soft music). The yoga practitioner will ensure that your breathing is controlled. You carry out the exercises in a very slow and controlled manner with your body in alignment. There are several different branches of yoga, each taking you to a different level.

Can yoga help dyslexia and ADHD?

Yoga is said to help people with learning difficulties, including dyslexia and ADHD, by facilitating deep relaxation, development of body awareness, memory and concentration and balance control. Yogic eye exercises are said to particularly benefit people with dyslexia and other learning difficulties by strengthening the optic nerve and stimulating various centres of the brain.

How many classes are needed?

This type of therapy is usually held at your local gym, health club or yoga centre. Many people attend on a weekly basis and say they feel wonderfully relaxed and refreshed.

Who will benefit most?

Yoga can assist a wide range of conditions, including stress reductions, eliminating tension, retaining and regaining movement, increasing muscle tone, slowing down the heart rate and decreasing blood pressure.

Can this be done at home?

Yoga can easily be carried out at home. There are many DVDs and videos available (see Resources).

Pilates

Pilates was developed by a German refugee, Joseph Pilates, who migrated to America. Although many of us think of Pilates as one of the latest fitness trends it has been in existence since the 1920s. Pilates, developed a set of exercises that work the deep core muscles of the torso and back, helping to affect the overall ability of range and motion of the body. By strengthening these muscle groups, they increase flexibility and help prevent back injuries. To aid this technique, Pilates also developed an assortment of different machines with names like the 'Reformer' and the 'Cadillac', which work in conjunction with his methods. There are two ways to work with Pilates: Mat Classes or in a dedicated Pilates studio with specialized equipment.

How do Pilates practitioners work?

The Pilates method uses exercises performed on a mat or using specialist equipment. These specialist exercise machines are said to work the whole body. Many of the machines use cables and trolleys (and unusual body positioning). The exercises stretch and lengthen the muscles to encourage coordination to stabilize the body.

When attending a Pilates class, the practitioner will ensure that your breathing is controlled. You carry out the exercises in a very slow and controlled manner and your body is in alignment. An important part of this exercise method is to pay particular attention to your concentration. Pilates practitioners believe that concentration triggers the brain to 'pay attention'. Pilates techniques are said to be used by many professional dancers, who find them an effective way to improve body awareness and alignment.

The Pilates Mat Class is a relatively new form of Pilates using mats on which to perform the exercises and stretches. It is similar to a yoga class, with the emphasis on physical change through breathing and posture, rather than spiritual development.

How many classes are needed?

This type of therapy is usually held at your local gym or health club. Many people find a Pilates class fun and attend each week.

Who will benefit most?

Practitioners consider it useful for many types of conditions including overcoming learning difficulties and improving coordination. It is also said to be excellent for dancers, models, and other artistic performers.

Can this be done at home?

Pilates can easily be carried out at home. There are a number of DVDs and videos available (see Resources).

Feldenkrais

Feldenkrais (rhymes with rice) was developed by a Russian-born Israeli scientist, Moshe Feldenkrais. He was an athlete and when his doctors couldn't restore full movement to an injured knee he started to look at his knowledge of anatomy, physics and psychology to heal his problems. The method is a unique approach to movement through re-education and aims to improve your physical and mental functioning by making you aware of how you move. The method become popular in the 1970s and is similar to other mind–body therapies, including the Alexander technique.

The Feldenkrais method is a unique approach to movement re-education and focuses on how movement is organized by the neuromuscular system. Feldenkrais therapists do not attempt to structurally alter the body. There are two components to this method. The first component, Functional Integration (FI), which is hands-on, involves the client lying on a table, sitting or standing while the practitioner uses touch to manipulate their muscles and joints, to help them sense and improve their movement patterns.

The second component, Awareness Through Movement (ATM), is taught verbally. Clients lie down, sit or stand and are guided through movement sequences. The emphasis is on slow, non-aerobic movement. These are usually group lessons.

Practitioners consider the two components to be equivalent, complementary ways of achieving the same results. Loose, comfortable clothing is worn for both. The Feldenkrais method does not treat or cure clients. It is seen as a supportive therapy and consists of a series of sessions rather than treatments.

How many sessions are needed?

Usually Feldenkrais therapy is offered in four to six sessions of about 45 minutes.

Who will benefit most?

Practitioners consider it useful for many types of chronic pain, as well as neuromuscular disorders, cerebral palsy, mobility. It is also beneficial for improving balance (dyspraxia), coordination and dyslexia. It is considered useful to dancers and other performers.

Can this be done at home?

This therapy can easily be used at home, once the client understands how it works.

Zero Balancing

Zero Balancing was devised in 1973 by an American physician and osteopath, Dr Fritz Smith. It is a healing treatment that works to align a person's body and energy with the body's physical structure, thereby optimizing health and physical fitness. This relatively new therapy often uses practitioners with osteopathy or chiropractic training.

How does it work?

Zero Balancing therapists work on the premise that since bones are the densest tissue in the body they hold the most energy. Practitioners work on the body's physical structure to release energy stored in the bones – release the energy and it will have a ripple effect throughout the body. Smith recognized and mapped out energy pathways around certain points on the body. These energy pathways are called pivotal points. Zero Balancing therapists have been trained to recognize these pivotal points and will always follow the same pattern during the therapy.

As the client lies fully clothed on a table, the practitioner will start to press gently but firmly onto the pivotal points of the hips, legs, along the spine, the neck, feet and head. Whilst the therapist is doing this they are checking the energy flow. By working on specific areas of the body they release the tension around these areas, thereby bringing energy and structure into balance.

How many sessions are needed?

As with any alternative therapy, treatment time varies, but usually clients have three or four sessions to begin the practice, and then may return for another session every few weeks.

Who will benefit most?

Zero Balancing helps with any condition caused by stress or an energetic imbalance.

Summing up

The therapies in this chapter are probably the most well known in alternative and/or complimentary areas. These therapies have been around for a long time and stood the test of time. Many therapists in this field work alongside the medical profession using natural and holistic methods to help strengthen the immune system. Because they are so well known and many doctors refer clients to them, many people find it a good way to start using alternative therapies. For useful addresses, please go to p.122.

Chapter 5

DEVELOPMENTAL DELAY

Movement-based therapists believe that learning difficulties can be caused by immature (primitive) reflexes remaining in the body. Attainment of balance, hand–eye coordination, motor control and perceptual skills may be delayed or inhibited as a result. There has been a lot of research in recent years to show that some children with these problems can be helped with a movement-based programme (see, for example, Koester and Sherwood 2001; Blythe 2005). There are now a significant number of therapies with different types of exercise programmes, ranging from simple exercises to working with looking at flashing lights on computers, or rolling around the floor like a baby. The list includes:

- Brain Gym®
- Primary Movement®
- Learning Breakthrough
- Brushing technique.

Brain Gym®

Brain Gym® was developed in the 1970s by Paul Dennison PhD, a remedial educational specialist, to help children and adults overcome learning difficulties through physical movement. It is sometimes referred to as Educational Kinesiology (Edu-K). Brain Gym® is the registered trademark for an Educational Kinesiology.

The programme consists of 26 physical movements that enhance learning and performance, by developing the brain's neural pathways through movement. These activities came about from Dennison's knowledge of the relationship of movement to perception, and the impact on fine motor and academic skills. The programme works on the physical rather than mental components of learning.

How does it work?

Dennison produced 26 exercises that he called the Three Dimensions:

- Laterality – the ability to coordinate one side of the brain with the other. This skill is fundamental to the ability to read, write, and communicate.

- Focus – the ability to coordinate the back and front areas of the brain. It is related to comprehension, the ability to find meaning and to experience details within their context.

- Centring – the ability to coordinate the top and bottom areas of the brain. This skill is related to organization, grounding, feeling and expressing one's emotions, a sense of personal space.

Clients following a movement programme carry out a number of these exercises on a daily basis. The activities reinforce positive movement and postural habits. Eventually these movements become automatic and help develop fine motor skills.

The activities have names that appeal to young children such as the Owl, the Elephant, Alphabet 8s and the Lazy Eight Track. All the exercises work on slightly different areas of the body. For example, the Lazy Eight Track is said to integrate complex neuropathways, improving visual focus, tracing and reading comprehension. The activity is carried out using a marble. With your finger you follow the marble along the 'curve' of the figure eight (which is carved out on a wooden board). This movement enhances fine motor control, which is claimed to help literacy skills.

Can Brain Gym® help dyslexia and ADHD?

Brain Gym® practitioners consider it particularly useful for many types of learning difficulties, especially dyspraxia, ADHD and dyslexia, by improving concentration, memory, reading, writing, organization, physical and coordination problems.

Who will benefit most?

Brain Gym® is used in more than 80 countries worldwide. It is taught in many schools and performing arts colleges and used in athletic training programmes.

Can this be done at home?

Brain Gym® activities can be carried out at home once a programme has been set up. A good introductory book is available, *Brain Gym®: Simple Activities for Whole Brain Learning* (Dennison and Dennison 1992).

Primary Movement®

The Primary Movement® programme was developed at Queen's University Belfast, Northern Ireland. It is a unique movement programme which works on the premise that children with specific reading difficulties have problems with balance and motor control. They look at persistent primary reflexes, which are linked in the earliest months of life to balance. It is suggested that children who still have these primary reflexes beyond the usual time could indicate developmental delay, which has been linked to learning difficulties. The organization works to promote training courses and other facilities for those working with children with specific learning difficulties.

How does it work?

Primary Movement® promotes early intervention through movement for children with specific learning difficulties. Primary reflexes are said to be critical for the survival of the newborn, for example, grasping and infant rooting, sucking reflexes. There are said to be more than 70 primary reflexes.

Primary Movement® is considered helpful for people with dyslexia by carrying out special movements and exercises. It is suggested that these techniques could easily be implemented into a physical education lesson in schools.

Primary Movement® therapists believe that many children with dyslexia and other learning difficulties still have strong primary reflexes that are hindering their ability to do normal age-related activities such as holding a pencil or drawing a straight line. Primary Movement® uses exercise and movements to mimic these reflexes and switch them off, thereby promoting coordination. It is these special routines, which are designed to improve reflexes, that in turn lead to improved literacy skills.

Can Primary Movement® help dyslexia and ADHD?

Primary Movement® practitioners consider it useful for many types of learning difficulties, including dyslexia and ADHD.

Can it be done at home?

Once set up, exercise programmes can easily be followed at home.

Learning Breakthrough

In the 1960s Dr Frank Belgau, director of the Visual and Motor Perception Lab at the University of Houston, began experimenting with children who had high IQs but were having difficulty reading. Belgau found that using balancing exercises improved the reading ability of his clients. He first published the Learning Breakthrough Program™ in 1982 (Belgau and Belgau 1982).

The Learning Breakthrough Program™ is a balance and sensory activity programme designed to help better organize brain processing in order to improve a child's overall functioning in areas of learning such as reading, writing, comprehension and focus. This exercise-based programme is said to stimulate sensory integration, spatial awareness and sense of balance.

How does it work?

There are several different therapists trained to use this programme, including occupational therapists, developmental optometrists, speech therapists, audiologists, teachers and parents.

The Learning Breakthrough Program™ involves clients watching a video recording that takes him through tasks which include throwing beanbags, tossing balls at a 'bounce back target' and tapping a hanging ball while standing on a balance board. The method uses balance and sensory activities on a daily basis. The activities are said to have a positive effect on brain processes involved in learning, balance, dexterity and motor skills.

How many sessions are needed?

To see permanent change it is advisable that the programme is followed consistently twice a day for 15 minutes for a period of 9 to 12 months.

The programme can be used in a group setting as well as one-to-one therapy.

Who will benefit most?

The Learning Breakthrough Program™ is suitable for anyone over the age of seven years. It is said to help a wide range of learning difficulties, including reading difficulties, clumsiness, low self-esteem, handwriting problems, dyspraxia, dyslexia, ADHD, etc. It is claimed that this programme not only helps clients to catch up but may also benefit gifted children.

Can this be done at home?

This programme comes complete with equipment, instruction manual and demonstrated on VHS or DVD (see Useful addresses for ordering details). The Learning Breakthrough Program™ can be carried out at home or in a school environment without the need for specific training.

Brushing technique by David Mulhall

Brushing is a treatment that can be used with children and adults. In terms of unlocking developmental delay or learning difficulties it is unusual in its claim to deal with retained early (foetal) reflexes and not just primitive (infant) reflexes. It is based on the belief that, as neuro-physiological development begins in the womb, it is crucial to be able to access the earliest stages of the developmental process to ensure a successful outcome.

It recognizes early and primitive reflexes as the underlying cause of learning difficulties (which has nothing to do with lack of intelligence or ability, quite the opposite). The technique asserts that if these reflexes are retained beyond infancy they will cause developmental delay in childhood and later life, holding back academic achievement, physical dexterity, coordination, emotional and social maturity, speech and language skills as well as neuro-acoustic ability. Higher adrenalin levels (hyperactivity) are also common among the children and adults attending this treatment.

It aims to assess at what stage neuro-physiological developmental delay has occurred through physical testing. For example, a seven-year-old boy who is extremely good at chess struggles to read. An 11-year-old girl with excellent physical coordination has the vocabulary and verbal skills of a child of eight. A 37-year-old man with limited powers of concentration finds reading a chore. It is not a question of being stupid or lazy; the problem is that they are stuck at a much earlier age in certain aspects of their development.

The examples above illustrate in very simple terms how retained primitive and early reflexes wreak havoc with the developmental process and long-term prospects of individuals. There is no rhyme or reason and unfortunately some of us have a much tougher time than others. The disparity between potential and performance confuses parents, teachers and employers alike. In boys, the warning signs manifest themselves earlier on – boys age seven to eight form the majority of my clients. Girls, on the other hand, generally cope better in the primary school years, then plateau with the onset of puberty and sometimes develop emotional problems. Symptoms can manifest themselves across the board (global developmental delay) or in a fairly limited way (when a child displays classic dyslexic traits only) but things are never clear-cut.

What has become more and more clear in my work over the last ten years is the significant detrimental impact that retained primitive and early reflexes also have on a person's general well-being and consequently on family life. Developmental delay does not confine itself to the traditional symptoms of learning difficulties. There are other less well-known associated symptoms that make life much harder than it needs to be for the adult and child. Bedwetting or soiling over the age of five is likely to indicate that the bladder or sphincter is being controlled by muscle tension alone, resulting in accidents. A poor appetite or picky eating often suggests an immature digestive system. An exercise-mad workaholic husband or wife who can't relax even on holiday is producing too much adrenalin (hyperactivity). Hyper-sensitivity (severe physical discomfort in response to light touching, hair or nail cutting and wearing certain fabrics) is another indicator of developmental delay. Eczema, rashes, migraine and asthma are other common factors but these conditions fade away during treatment.

Stimulating specific nerve endings through brushing kick-starts the develop-mental process once again. It activates outdated reflexes in order to shut them down, enabling the child or adult to evolve, while at the same time developing the vital postural reflexes that we need and depend on for the rest of our lives. What we need to understand is that development never stops: it is a continuing lifelong process. What we need to grasp is that there is a way of smoothing out the neuro-physiological glitches picked up along the way. It is never too late to make life easier for ourselves, our children, and perhaps most importantly our grandchil-dren. Developmental delay sometimes exists in families for generations. Brushing has the potential to break the chain.

Assessment

Further information on the Brushing technique can be obtained from the David Mulhall Centre (see Useful addresses section).

Summing up

Therapists working in this field believe that learning difficulties can be caused by immature (primitive) reflexes remaining in the body leading to learning difficulties, especially with literacy skills.

Many of these therapists use movement-based exercises to increase children's mobility. Many therapists support the theory that children can be helped by going back to basics – crawling, rolling over etc., which is claimed will help to develop these underdeveloped areas. Some of the therapies have shown good results. However, as with other therapies mentioned in this book, some of these can cost a great deal of money and there is usually no money back guarantee. For useful addresses, please go to p.122.

Chapter 6

VISION

Over recent years there have been many studies to show that children with undiagnosed eye problems often have learning difficulties (Eden, Stein, Wood *et al.* 1995). It stands to reason if a child cannot see properly they will not be able to read, spell and write. Therefore, it is important that all children have eye tests during infancy and preschool years and then annually to detect any problems at the earliest opportunity.

There are a significant number of related therapies with different types of tests to help you. These range from vision training to working with computers or 'putting a hat on a donkey' (Dunlop test). The list covers:

- Irlen Syndrome
- Coloured overlays
- Intuitive Colorimeter
- ChromaGen™ lenses
- Harris Filters
- Visual Tracking Magnifier
- Dunlop test
- Optometric evaluation.

I have included a short vision checklist to help identify whether the child actually does have a vision problem. If your child has more than a few of the signs or symptoms listed, it would be advisable to make an appointment with an orthoptist before investigating further.

Vision checklist

When reading, does your child:

- hold the book a few inches from his face?
- close one eye in order to see better?
- skip over or omit words?
- use a finger or bookmark to help keep his place?
- complain of blurred vision?
- reverse letters or numbers?
- complain of print 'running together'?
- complain of words 'wobbling about'?
- complain of double vision?
- complain of headaches?
- excessively rub or blink his eyes?
- frown, scowl or squint?
- suffer from excessive tiredness after close work?

When spelling, does your child:

- have difficulties?
- spell correctly and later spell it wrong?
- learn spellings well for tests, but then forget?
- transpose letters in words?

When writing, does your child:

- write letters back to front?
- write letters backwards in writing?

If you would like to investigate vision therapies further, then perhaps check out the following therapies.

Irlen Syndrome

In 1983 an American psychologist, Helen Irlen, discovered a perceptual problem caused by light sensitivity. This syndrome is called Irlen Syndrome and is a type of visual perceptual problem. The syndrome has also been called Scotopic Sensitivity Syndrome (SSS), Visual Dyslexia and Asfedia. It is not an optical problem, but a problem with how the nervous system encodes and decodes visual information.

What is Irlen Syndrome?

Irlen found that individuals with Irlen Syndrome saw the printed page differently from those with normal vision. She found that some students benefited from the use of coloured overlays. The specially formulated coloured overlays or coloured lenses worn as spectacles or contact lenses appear to work by filtering out light that causes distortions to print on paper. The problems appeared to be worse with black print on white paper.

What happens when you go for a test?

The orthoptist will use a variety of tests, including reading.

Can I have coloured spectacles?

You can have spectacles or contact lenses.

Who will benefit most?

Irlen Syndrome is thought to affect about 50% of students with specific learning difficulties such as dyslexia. You may benefit from spectacles or lenses if when reading you find:

- letters merge together
- letters appear in the wrong order
- letters twirl
- words are fuzzy
- words jump about
- difficulties in reading and keeping your place
- excessive rubbing and blinking of eyes
- words appear as a jumbled puzzle
- words appear faded.

Coloured overlays

Some people say that when they use coloured plastic sheets over their work they are able to read more easily. These plastic sheets may help people with dyslexia and other specific learning difficulties. Coloured overlays are transparent coloured vinyl sheets that can be placed over a page in a book. They work by reducing the perceptual distortions of text (some students say the words go fuzzy or jump about.) These signs are characteristic of a condition known as Meares-Irlen Syndrome or Scotopic Sensitivity Syndrome (SSS).

How does it work?

Some students with dyslexia and/or specific learning difficulties say they find it easier to read more fluently and quickly when using overlays. They can read faster, for longer and do not get as tired. The overlays may also help to improve comprehension.

The sheets are available in different colours and students should try them to see which ones they feel most comfortable with. If after a period of time the student receives a continued benefit, spectacles can be made in order that they may use them in other areas of their work. If you are working on a computer you may benefit from changing the colour on your screen.

It is important to note that lenses in spectacles will usually be different colours from the coloured overlays because of the difference in the distance between the text and the colour film.

Who will benefit most?

Some students with dyslexia have reported that they can read more quickly and easily and more fluently when using overlays.

Where can I find someone to test me?

These eye tests can be carried out at participating opticians and usually offer both coloured overlay trials and the supply of colour-corrected optical tinting in accordance with the Cerium Optics standards. Participating opticians have an Intuitive Colorimeter for accurate assessment of the effectiveness of the overlay hues.

It is usually advisable to have a full eye examination when being assessed as this can often reveal other previously undiagnosed visual problems.

Where can I get coloured overlays?

If you suspect someone may have a problem in the first instance, Cerium Overlays are a logical and inexpensive first step towards assessment. The Cerium Overlays and Screening Kit can be purchased through Cerium Visual Technologies.

Intuitive Colorimeter

Some people say that when they use colour in their spectacles they have been able to read more easily. These spectacles are made with the help of the Intuitive Colorimeter and may help people with dyslexia and other specific learning difficulties.

The Intuitive Colorimeter is a machine developed by the Medical Research Council and manufactured under licence by Cerium Visual Technologies Ltd. In order to determine the tint, an assessment is carried out using the Intuitive Colorimeter to assess exactly which colour is needed for the individual. The Intuitive Colorimeter uses up to 7000 tints to measure exactly which colour may help.

How does it work?

Scientists do not know exactly how this technique works but they believe that the area in the brain that controls vision is very sensitive and some text may overexcite the colour neurones resulting in text being distorted. For instance, people with dyslexia seem to be affected by striped patterns (including the striped lines of text). Some people find it difficult to read because of the glare from white paper, which in turn leads to eyestrain and headaches. It appears that coloured lenses filter out light and stop the glare, helping to correct the problem.

Who will benefit most?

Students who appear to benefit most from these lenses are those who find that words and letters tend to be jumbled up, move around, wobble and appear in the wrong order. Some students with dyslexia and/or specific learning difficulties may have most of the following symptoms, whereas others may only have one. Mostly, students do not realize it is a problem as they have always seen writing in the same way. Some people who have used coloured overlays claim to have noticed an increase in their reading speed and fewer headaches.

Where can I find someone to test me?

The full screening test using the Intuitive Colorimeter is available through participating optometrists.

ChromaGen™ lenses

Some students say that when they wear special contact lenses that have a tiny speck of colour they have been able to read more easily. These contact lenses are made with the help of the Intuitive Colorimeter and may help people with dyslexia and other specific learning difficulties. ChromaGen™ lenses were originally developed at the Corneal Laser Centre for colour blindness at Clattersbridge Hospital, Wirral.

How does it work?

ChromaGen™ lenses are similar to ordinary soft contact lenses but have a tiny speck of colour that is almost invisible. This speck of colour is usually tinted with a variety of filters of a specific density and hue, and it appears in the circle covering the black part of the eye (the pupil). These filters have been so successful that it is now possible to have spectacles made with the filters in, like a 'one-way mirror'.

Who will benefit most?

Professor John Stein, a neuroscientist at Oxford University, has estimated that approximately one in three people who have dyslexia could suffer from the visual form that can be helped by special coloured filters (BBC News, 2nd July 2003).

Will ChromaGen™ lenses help dyslexia and ADHD?

It is claimed that ChromaGen™ lenses can help with a wide range of learning difficulties, including dyslexia, dyspraxia and ADD (with or without hyperactivity).

Where can I find someone to test me?

Assessments are available through licensed practitioners. For further information, contact Cantor & Nissel (see Useful addresses).

Harris Filters

In 1996 David Harris invented the lenses that are now marketed by a contact lens manufacturer as ChromaGen™ lenses. Harris continued researching for solutions to help people with dyslexia. His dedicated work using special filters led to the recent development of the filter technology called Harris Filters. The Harris Filter technology is now well known and widely used in the UK and USA.

Will these lenses help dyslexia?

Many people with dyslexia report problems when reading such as losing their place, reading the same piece over and over again, blurred letters or letters that 'wobble about'. Harris Filters are special lenses that work by reducing visual perceptual distortions and are said to help by reducing or eliminating these visual perceptions. It is claimed that Harris Filters can help people with dyslexia to improve performance and make reading easier.

Where can I find someone to test me?

Assessments can only be performed by a practitioner at a Harris Foundation clinic (see Useful addresses).

Visual Tracking Magnifier

The Visual Tracking Magnifier (VTM) was developed after many years of research by Ian Jordan, who is well known for his pioneering work in designing equipment that can effectively measure and help visual dyslexia.

Many visual dyslexia sufferers are confused by pattern glare, which causes whole blocks of text to merge and swim above the page, making reading extremely difficult. Jordan has combated this problem by creating a device that modifies the way one's eyes approach the print. A useful book about visual problems is *Visual Dyslexia – A Guide for Parents & Teachers* (Jordan 2002).

How does it work?

The VTM sits on a page and can be easily tracked backwards and forwards across the text. It consists of a high-powered magnifying glass, with a central viewing strip about one centimetre wide. Above and below this strip are two semi-circular, transparent, patterned areas that remove any distortion of the surrounding text. As a result, a high proportion of visual dyslexics can read text much more easily.

Who will benefit most?

Some people find that when reading they have difficulties keeping their place on a line of text. The VTM product is very useful for this particular problem.

Where can I get a VTM?

The Visual Tracking Magnifier is available from Edward Marcus Ltd (see Useful addresses).

Dunlop test

The Dunlop test was designed in 1971 by Mrs P. Dunlop, an orthoptist, to ascertain whether a child has a fixed reference eye (or lead eye). If the reference eye (lead eye) is not established this could create learning difficulties.

How does it work?

If your child has an eye problem he may be referred to an eye clinic. An orthoptist will assess his binocular vision to see how his eyes work together and to make sure he has a fixed reference eye. The orthoptist will carry out various tests to ascertain whether the child's visual problems are associated with learning problems.

The Dunlop test involves looking into a special machine at pictures that help to decide which eye is in charge of sending a message, in the form of a picture, to the language centre in the brain to decipher what the picture (i.e. word) says. It is a two-eyed test. Both eyes are open – to ascertain whether a reference or lead eye is established. This should not be confused with a dominant eye which is tested when you hold a tube or kaleidoscope to one eye – invariably the other eye is automatically closed.

Who will benefit most?

Children usually have a fixed reference eye by the time they are seven years old. If treatment is necessary, spectacles with one side frosted or eye exercises may be prescribed.

Are special spectacles needed?

Some people are prescribed spectacles with one lenses frosted over, other people are sometimes given exercises to do.

Where can I find someone to test me?

The Dunlop test is usually carried out in the orthoptic departments of participating hospitals.

Optometric evaluation by Keith Holland

In order to be able to concentrate, absorb information and maintain interest in the written word, the visual system of a young person needs certain capabilities. The eyes have to be capable of moving smoothly and easily along a line of print, jumping back and down to the beginning of the next line and repeating this action for extended periods of time. Students also have to be able to adjust the focus of their eyes rapidly from distance to near and back again when copying from a black-board.

Conscious or subconscious?

It is important that these activities can be performed without conscious thought or effort. If the brain has to 'use up' concentration and energy in order simply to move the eyes along a line of print, then there is less likelihood that the contents of the text will have any meaning that will be remembered, or that the words coming next will be anticipated. Reading has to become a subconscious action.

Learning to read

Learning to move the eyes in a way that enables us to read efficiently is, like changing gear, a learned action. Some young people fail to develop this skill and as a result their reading and writing abilities are often lower than expected.

Other skills such as ball catching or graceful gymnastic body movements can also be affected and children with poorly developed vision systems are frequently observed to be clumsy and ill-coordinated.

Behaviour optometry

Some fully qualified and state registered optometrists now additionally practise what is called behaviour optometry. Behaviour optometrists operate on the basis that visual skills are learned and therefore trainable. Vision is considered to be an inseparable part of the whole human system and should not be regarded as a separate and individual function. This means that our behaviour and environment can influence the way in which our visual system works, and vice versa. Behavioural optometrists use activities and training to improve the efficiency of the whole visual system.

Vision training

Vision training, or vision therapy, provides a means of learning to use the visual system in a more efficient manner. When the visual system works more efficiently, more information can be received, processed and understood. When there are problems with visual perception, achieving full potential can be helped by using the techniques of vision training. This involves developing good body bilaterality, hand–eye coordination, form perception, directionality and visualization skills, as well as ensuring that the muscles which focus and direct the eyes are functioning efficiently. Should vision training be necessary, these terms will become more meaningful as the therapy programme progresses.

Who can benefit?

Students with good visual abilities read faster with less effort, understand more of what they read and retain it longer. Athletes who use their vision effectively see things more quickly and more accurately and show good overall performance. The improvement in the processing of visual information can benefit many areas of life, especially at school, in sports and at work.

Optometric vision training is individually programmed to the specific needs of each patient, with the basic universally needed skills being included in all programmes. Other activities are designed to meet specific needs.

What to look for

Children who may benefit from vision training can often be seen when reading to have difficulty in keeping their place and in following lines of print. Typically a child will read with a finger or a marker under the line being read, and as they read they will move the whole of the head rather than simply following the print with their eyes. In many cases mathematical ability and intelligence may be normal or higher than normal for the age, and yet reading presents a problem.

The concentration span of a young person with a poorly developed visual system will often be very short, and time spent reading may come to an abrupt halt with sudden complete lack of interest.

Who can help?

Obviously if a child has learning difficulties all avenues of possible help have to be explored. In order to establish if there may be a visual component to the learning difficulty then a full eye examination must be carried out by an optometrist.

If it is suspected that there may be a developmental visual problem, in other words all the bits are there and healthy but are not coordinating properly, then your optometrist may wish to deal with this himself. Alternatively you may choose to be referred to a behavioural optometrist who has more experience in helping with learning problems.

The British Association of Behavioural Optometrists maintains a register of all optometrists who have attended a further education course specifically designed to develop their knowledge and skills.

Summing up

There are various tests for evaluating children's eye problems. Sometimes all that is required is just a quick and simple eye test. Others may need vision training or coloured spectacles may help. There is considerable choice now so it is up to you to decide. Vision training may seem quite complicated, but quite simply it means fully testing the eyes and training them to respond to appropriate treatment. This treatment may take a few months or several years but if successful it can be of great help to the child. For useful addresses please go to p.122.

Chapter 7

NUTRITION AND HEALTH

Most people would accept the premise that eating a balanced diet is essential to children's mental and physical development. A complete diet is necessary in the development of vision, learning ability and coordination. But are our children getting a well-balanced diet or should they be taking supplements? Can taking supplements of fatty acids, zinc and iron reduce the symptoms of dyslexia, dyspraxia and ADHD? Could deficiencies in these vital vitamins and minerals even cause dyslexia?

In 1981, the late Mrs I. Colquhoun and Mrs S. Bunday put forward a radical proposal to the medical profession suggesting a link between people with ADHD and a lack of fatty acids in their diet. They noted that children with hyperactivity or ADD often had other symptoms such as excessive thirst, dry skin and allergies. They carried out a survey of over 200 children with hyperactivity and concluded their problems were linked to biochemical imbalances. These were caused by deficiency of essential fatty acids. Two of these fatty acids are supplied by evening primrose oil and it was noted that there was an improvement in hyperactivity in children who took the oil. The scientific establishment, however, never took their claims seriously. Twenty years later, their findings were confirmed in the *American Journal of Clinical Nutrition* (Burgess *et al.* 2000). Further research has also supported their earlier findings that some children with dyslexia or ADHD can be helped with essential fatty acids (Richardson and Puri 2002).

Over the last three decades much research has been carried out into food and learning difficulties (Dewhurst *et al.* 2003; Konofal *et al.* 2004; Bruner *et al.* 1996). Some of the problems being looked at are:

- salicylates, food additives, colourings, flavourings
- refined sugar

- fatty acid deficiencies

- zinc deficiencies

- iron deficiencies

- herbal medicine

- Ayurvedic medicine

- food allergies, multiple chemical sensitivities.

Feingold Hypothesis

During the 1970s Dr Ben Feingold from California also put forward the idea that food was to blame for the rise in learning difficulties. The Feingold Hypothesis, as it is commonly referred to, claimed that many children with ADHD were sensitive to artificial food colours, flavourings and preservatives, and in particular to a group of chemicals called salicylates. When Feingold analysed the diets of hyperactive children he found many of them had high levels of these chemicals.

Many food additives contain salicylates, but they can also be found to occur naturally in food such as almonds, apples, brazil nuts, broccoli, carrots, grapes, oranges, tomatoes, yeast products, cola, coffee and tea. It has been shown that naturally occurring salicylates are not as harmful as the artificial ones. Initially it was thought that every hyperactive child was allergic to salicylates but it has emerged that in approximately 70% of cases food intolerance or true food allergy is to blame.

Refined sugar

Some specialists and parents believe that hyperactivity in children is made worse by excessive amounts of sugar in the diet. It is said that when we have too much sugar it can affect the immune system. Many hyperactive children eat a lot of junk food. If these junk foods, which are high in salt, refined carbohydrates and sugar, are replaced by complex carbohydrates or snacks containing protein, specialists believe that the behaviour of many hyperactive children would improve dramatically.

Fatty acids

Is a deficit in essential fatty acids to blame for the four-fold increase in dyslexia, dyspraxia, ADHD and other specific learning difficulties that we have seen over the last 20 years? There have been many studies that show that abnormal levels of fatty acids in the brain could be responsible for the practical and behavioural problems experienced by dyslexic children, as well as those with dyspraxia and attention deficit/hyperactivity disorder (ADHD) (Richardson 2002; Richardson and Puri 2000; Richardson and Puri 2002; Portwood 2002).

Some studies have shown that underachieving children have improved when their diets were supplemented with fish oils (Richardson and Montgomery 2005). The fish oils contain omega-3 fatty acids, which are essential for brain development and function but are largely missing from modern processed diets.

What are essential fatty acids?

Essential fatty acids (EFAs) play a major role in brain function. They are required for visual functioning in the retina of the eye, in the synapses of the brain, in nerve tissues and in the adrenals for regulating stress. However, EFAs cannot be synthesized by the body and must be provided through diet. The richest source of EFAs is said to be oily fish. Breast milk and formula milk provide some benefit for the developing baby.

It may be that the problem with modern diets is that they lack EFAs, perhaps because we are eating less fresh fish than our predecessors. EFAs are highly perishable (or biodegradable) and are therefore not found in many packaged and processed foods.

Fatty acids deficit checklist

This list will give you an idea whether your child (or you) could be deficient in essential fatty acids:

- excessive thirst
- rough dry skin
- dandruff
- soft/brittle nails
- dull or dry hair
- poor night vision
- sensitivity to bright light
- letters move, blur, wobble about or go fuzzy when reading
- poor concentration

- poor working memory
- mood swings
- sleep problems
- allergies
- tiredness
- dyslexia or other specific learning difficulties
- poor wound healing.

Can natural foods improve deficiency?

Many foods contain essential fatty acids including:

- oily fish, for example, anchovies, halibut, herring, mackerel, pilchards, salmon, sardines, fresh tuna, trout, turbot, whitebait
- seafood, including eels, New Zealand green lipped mussels, shark
- flax seeds or flax seed oil
- milk (organic)
- pumpkin seeds and oil
- rapeseed oil (canola oil)
- soybeans and soybean oil
- walnuts and walnut oil
- wheatgerm.

Research by the Institute of Grassland and Environmental Research in Wales has shown that organic milk contains two-thirds more omega-3 essential fatty acids than ordinary milk (Dewhurst *et al.* 2003).

People who do not want to take fish supplements can try flax seeds or flax seed oil, which are excellent sources of omega-3 EFAs.

Are there side effects from taking fish oils?

The companies selling fish oil supplements advise people to build up the dosage of pills slowly in order to avoid gastric intolerance. As fish oil is a natural and effective way of thinning the blood, care should be taken when used in conjunction with blood-thinning drugs (e.g. Warfarin) and advice should be obtained from your medical practitioner. If you are on any medication or if you intend to give supplements to children, you should always check first with your practitioner.

Where can I buy essential fatty acids?

Several products containing essential fatty acids are available, including Efalex® (liquid or tablets) and eye q®. These supplements are available from chemists, health shops and supermarkets.

Zinc deficiency

Zinc is one of the body's most important trace minerals and there have been some suggestions to indicate that people with dyslexia and other learning difficulties may be deficient in this mineral (Grant, Howard and Davies 1988).

Zinc is an essential mineral and plays an important part in the body's immune system. Zinc also helps to maintain fertility in adults, growth in children and boosts the immune system. A shortage can affect the healing process because the body is unable to store it. Therefore it is vital that we take enough in our daily diet to stay healthy.

How would I know if I was zinc deficient?

The most common symptoms of zinc deficiency are:

- lack of appetite
- skin problems
- white marks on fingernails
- dandruff
- loss of taste sensation
- tiredness.

Where can zinc be found?

Zinc can be found in many foods including:

- lean meat
- liver
- Cheddar cheese
- chicken

- eggs
- wholemeal breads, wheatgerm
- whole grain cereals
- dried beans (black-eyed peas)
- fish (particularly herrings)
- oysters
- tofu
- seafood.

I drink a lot of coffee – could I be zinc deficient?

Some people do not realize that zinc can be destroyed or blocked by various dietary items such as tannin (found in tea, coffee, alcohol), food colourings and additives.

If I eat a well-balanced diet will I be okay?

Some dieticians believe that the average diet is deficient in zinc, particularly vegetarian diets.

Will I be all right if I take a zinc supplement?

Apparently zinc inhibits copper absorption, which can lead to anaemia and lower cholesterol levels. Therefore it is sometimes suggested that a copper supplement should also be used. Before taking supplements of any kind you should always take advice from your medical practitioner.

Iron deficiency

There is research to indicate that even a minor deficiency in iron may weaken the immune system and impair general physical performance. Iron deficiency has also been implicated in a number of conditions including learning disabilities and ADHD.

A French study (Konofal *et al.* 2004) has identified a link between iron deficiency and ADHD. Fifty-three children with ADHD were tested at a hospital in Paris and 84% of them had abnormal iron levels compared to only 18% in a control group. The study suggests that iron supplements may be useful in treating ADHD.

An earlier study published in the *Lancet* (Bruner *et al.* 1996) found that teenage girls showed cognitive improvement when they were given iron supplements. Previous research appears to show that anaemia affects the mental abilities of children. Animal research has also suggested that iron deficiency is enough to change brain iron levels, which in turn alter the way neurotransmitters, behave in the brain.

It would appear that iron deficiency may contribute to hyperactivity in some children, but there is not sufficient research to give us a conclusive answer. The best way to ensure an adequate supply of iron is through diet. A diet rich in iron-containing foods is an excellent way to ensure that the correct level of iron is maintained.

What foods contain good sources of iron?

Iron can be found in many foods including:

- liver
- red meat
- poultry
- fish
- eggs
- nuts and seeds
- beans
- dark green leafy vegetables
- bread and fortified breakfast cereals.

How would I know if I was iron deficient?

The most common symptoms of iron deficiency are:

- dizziness
- lethargy
- tiredness.

Is there a test to show iron deficiency?

A serum ferritin test will indicate iron deficiency. Depending on the result, an iron supplement containing the appropriate amount of iron could be taken. Iron is not easily eliminated from the body so caution should be exercised concerning the dosage. Too much iron can be toxic. Before taking supplements of any kind you should always take advice from your medical practitioner.

Herbal medicine

Herbal medicine (sometimes referred to as herbalism) is the use of plants for their therapeutic or medicinal effects. The medicinal use of herbs is said to be as old as mankind itself. Traditional herbal medicine has been used by all cultures to cure all ills. The very first medicines were derived from plants because that was all that was available. The World Health Organization (WHO) estimates that four billion people, 80% of the world population, presently use herbal medicine for some aspect of healthcare.

How do herbs work?

Herbal medicines concentrate on balancing and strengthening the whole person and can be used to treat a wide number of conditions. Some herbs can contain up to 200 different active constituents. For example, meadowsweet contains salicylates (from which aspirin is derived), but it also contains chemicals that protect the stomach lining from damage caused by salicylates. While aspirin can cause gastric bleeding and ulcers, meadowsweet is used to reduce stomach acid and to treat gastric ulcers.

Can herbs help dyslexia or ADHD?

There are claims made for many different herbs in the alleviation of dyslexia and other learning difficulties, two of which are kava kava and valerian, both used to relieve stress and anxiety.

What happens if I see a herbalist?

At the first appointment the herbalist will take a full medical history and discuss present health conditions. You will be asked to keep a diary of everything you eat and drink before this consultation. The herbalist will then recommend supplements to take based on this information.

What type of conditions can herbs help?

Herbal medicine is useful for a wide range of conditions, including arthritis, high blood pressure, ADHD and dyslexia. Some herbs have reportedly been effective against the superbug MRSA (Warn 2004).

Can this be done at home?

Herbal products can easily be used in the home. The demand for them has grown substantially with the increase in alternative therapies. They can be found in most supermarkets, chemists and health shops.

Can herbal products be dangerous?

It is a common assumption that because herbs are natural they must be safe. People should always check with their doctors before taking supplements, especially if they are on any sort of medication, as some herbs can interfere with potency or counteract the drug.

Ayurvedic medicine

Ayurvedic medicine is a traditional holistic health therapy which relies heavily on herbal medicine products. It evolved on the Indian subcontinent between 3000 and 5000 years ago and it is estimated that over three-quarters of the population uses Ayurvedic medicine. Ayurveda means 'the science of life' (pronounced eye-ur-vee-dah or eye-ur-vee-dic). The main emphasis of this therapy is on the prevention of loss of harmony in the person and to regain it if disharmony has occurred.

Ayurvedic medicine uses several natural approaches including dietary recommendations, meditation, exercise, massage, herbal medicines, yoga and examination of lifestyle.

How does it work?

Like many alternative therapies, Ayurvedic doctors treat the whole body, not just the symptoms of a disease. Its principles are based on three underlying energies called doshas:

1. Vata is the 'air type'.

2. Pitta is 'fire energy'.

3. Kapha is the 'earth type'.

Each of these doshas controls different parts of the body's functions. Ayurvedic therapists believe everyone is made up of these three doshas and they should all be equal. If one is out of balance it can affect overall well-being. An Ayurvedic practitioner will look at the whole person and work out the best treatment. A variety of medicines and massage therapies is used in this therapy.

Who will benefit most?

Ayurvedic medicine is thought to help a wide variety of problems including addictions, weight loss, alcohol abuse, osteoarthritis, sciatica and chronic fatigue.

Can this be done at home?

Ayurvedic medicine can be easily used in the home. The use of these products has grown substantially with the increase in alternative therapies and they are available in many countries, including America and the UK.

Can Ayurvedic products be dangerous?

Some people are concerned about the high levels of lead, mercury and arsenic contained in some Ayurvedic products.

Allergies and multiple chemical sensitivities
Are allergies to blame for the rise in learning problems?

Some parents and professionals believe that diet can exacerbate if not cause dyslexia, ADHD and similar learning difficulties. Eating habits and dietary choice have undergone profound change in the last 40 years. So many additives and preservatives are now placed in food that it is not surprising that they have an effect on the behaviour and health of children. The air is becoming polluted by fumes and chemicals and there is some suggestion that lead in petrol may be the cause of hyperactivity in children. During the 1970s UK schools started to have problems with pupils' behaviour and many children were labelled as dyslexic or ADHD.

Many of us understand that children can be allergic to milk, wheat etc., but it is now known that house dust, plastic, petrol fumes, household chemicals and the like can also cause severe reactions and lead to learning difficulties. Allergies can seriously affect the brain and nervous system. There is a strong relationship between allergies, dyslexia, ADHD and other specific learning difficulties. Some specialists think that before we label children as being dyslexic, ADHD or similar they should be routinely checked for allergies.

There is growing evidence to suggest that the old mantra 'we are what we eat' is truer today than ever before. But what are we to do? We can try to eat more healthily and eliminate junk food, but if the very air we breathe may be harming us then what is the answer?

If you think that your child could be suffering from some sort of allergy, before embarking on testing (which can be expensive) it might be helpful to take three steps:

1. Eliminate all junk food from the diet.

2. Reduce sugar intake.

3. Ensure the diet contains enough fatty acids.

If junk food is eliminated, sugar reduced and an adequate amount of fatty acids included, an improvement should be seen. However, this improvement may take a few months to manifest itself so do not expect a child's behaviour to change overnight.

Multiple chemical sensitivities

Some people consider that a new allergy exists called 'multiple chemical sensitivities', which is thought to be caused by an intolerance to certain chemicals found in the everyday environment. This is sometimes called, environmental illness, ecological illness, total allergy syndrome or bio-ecological illness.

Some doctors say that multiple chemical sensitivities are not true allergies. Although this is technically correct, we know these sensitivities are the result of a malfunction of the immune system. Symptoms can be as diverse as the traditional nasal stuffiness, wheezing etc., to musculoskeletal aches and pains. However, perhaps the most surprising symptoms relate to behaviour: confusion, inability to concentrate, hyperactivity and dyslexia. No one is quite sure how many people are affected by this problem but it could be that many more are suffering without being aware of it. Therefore, it is in everyone's best interests to limit the use of chemicals wherever possible.

How can I find out if my child is allergic to something?

The next step to identify an allergy would be testing. There are numerous tests available, from simple hair analyses to thorough blood tests. The list includes:

•   auricular cardiac reflex (ACR)

•   blood tests

- cytotoxic testing
- electrical testing
- elimination diet
- hair mineral analysis
- intradermal testing
- kinesiology – muscle testing
- sublingual drop testing
- Nambudripad's Allergy Elimination Technique (NAET)
- Jaffe-Mellor Technique (JMT).

Summing up

It is nearly 30 years since a link was found between food (especially fatty acid deficiencies) and specific learning difficulties, particularly ADHD (Colquhoun and Bunday 1981). It is about time that all children displaying learning difficulties were routinely tested before being labelled and put on drugs. For useful addresses, please go to p.122.

Chapter 8

THE POWER OF TOUCH

The power of touch is something we are all aware of and it can be used in so many different situations. All the therapies listed here work in a holistic and natural way to promote good health, strengthen the immune system, help flush out toxins and provide stimulation and relaxation.

Massage therapy is often seen as a holistic approach and many massage therapists work alongside medical professionals and often doctors refer clients to them. There are a significant number of related 'touch therapies' with different methods to help you including:

- massage
- acupressure
- acupuncture
- aromatherapy
- reflexology
- Reiki
- Bowen Technique
- Emotional Freedom Technique.

Massage

Massage is something we do automatically; if you have a headache you rub your temple and if you knock your elbow you rub it. With remedial massage, specific movements can help break down scar tissue and adhesions as well as having a beneficial effect on the muscles, circulation and nervous system. There are many health benefits to a massage. It is a holistic and natural way to promote good health. It strengthens the immune system, helps flush out toxins and provides stimulation.

How does it work?

The therapist will ask about medical background before they start treatment. Depending on what type of massage is being given, usually the client lies fully or partly unclothed on a table. Massage therapists claim to improve circulation; reduce inflammation and swelling; break down scar tissue; increase muscle tone; alleviate tension and high blood pressure, and promote a sense of well-being.

Can massage help dyslexia?

Massage is said to help with people with dyslexia by improving coordination and providing a calmer environment for learning. The Coordination and Massage Programme for Dyslexia and Learning has recently been set up in the UK to investigate and work with massage and clients with dyslexia.

Can massage help infants?

With the growing use of alternative and complementary therapies, the International Association of Infant Massage has been set up to help the growing number of parents seeking to look at infant massage and how it can help their children (see Useful addresses).

Are there different types of massage?

There are a number of types of massage. However, they all work to the same principle – to relax the client. The list includes:

- general massage (most well known)
- remedial massage: skilled treatment of the soft tissue to help ease muscular aches and pains
- Indian head massage: Ayurvedic massage which covers the upper back, upper arms, shoulders, neck, scalp and face and is particularly effective in relieving stress
- coordination and massage: programme for dyslexia and learning
- infant massage: strengthens the developing immune system and provides sensory stimulation.

How many sessions are needed?

As with any treatment, time varies but usually clients have three or four sessions to begin the practice and then some may come back for another session every few weeks.

Who will benefit most?

Massage has been used to good effect on a variety of conditions including backache, circulation problems, stress-related problems, dyslexia and/or hyperactivity.

Acupressure

Acupressure is a traditional Chinese medicine that was developed over 5000 years ago. It deals with the human body and the flow of natural energy within the body. It addresses the flow of ki/chi energy circulating along 12 major pathways called meridians which are linked to specific parts of the body. It is believed that these energy channels have points (acupoints) and they may become blocked. Each point is named first for the meridian it lies on, for example, the stomach meridian, lung meridian, bladder meridian, and then for its position along that line: lung six means this energy point is at the sixth point on the lung meridian. Targeting these points can release energy blocks and relieve pain. Acupressure is similar to acupuncture, but it uses the pressure of the fingers and hands instead of needles. Acupressure is an effective and gentle alternative to acupuncture.

How does it work?

Using firm pressure, the therapist works on the acupoints with the thumbs, fingers or hands by using a mixture of rubbing, vibration and kneading. This releases the blocked energy at the acupoints, allowing the body/mind to relax, and relieves pain. It also leads to improved circulation and stimulates blood tissues. Therapists say that if the energy pathways are blocked, this could manifest as frustration and irritability or on a physical level as pain or discomfort.

Who will benefit most?

Therapists working in the field say it is an effective preventative treatment for tension-related ailments. It can help with a wide range of disorders including ADD, anxiety and dyslexia by releasing tension in the body. It has also been found to be beneficial for pain, joint problems, gastric disorders and insomnia.

How many sessions are needed?

As with any alternative treatment, time varies but it would appear that people usually have three or four sessions for an hour at a time. Some people return regularly for therapy to keep the body's energies balanced.

Are there different acupressure methods?

There are a number of types of acupressure methods. However, they all work to the same principle of clearing out energy blockages and aiming to bring the body's energy flow back into balance. The list includes:

- acupressure (most well known)

- shiatsu, meaning 'finger pressure', uses a variety of massage techniques together with assisted exercise and stretching

- seitai is a combination of acupressure, manipulative and nutritional therapy.

Acupuncture

Acupuncture is an ancient oriental healing art, which was developed over 2500 years ago. Originally stone needles were used and later bronze, gold and silver needles. Nowadays, therapists use stainless steel needles which are sterilized and disposable. Acupuncture deals with the human body and the flow of natural energy within the body. These energy channels, known as meridians, have points (acupoints) which may become blocked. A therapist places needles in various acupoints on the body's surface. These help to break up energy blockages and return the organs etc. to good health. Acupuncture is a holistic system that attempts to restore the whole body to good health. Acupuncture is similar to acupressure but uses tiny needles instead of manual pressure.

How does it work?

Before you start treatment, acupuncturists will require a full medical history and a physical examination. They look not only at obvious physical symptoms but also at factors such as colour of skin, tone of voice, and in particular the conditions of the tongue, which is believed to reflect the overall health of the body. Acupuncturists also focus on the pulse, which is considered to be another major indicator of a client's overall condition.

Approximately ten to twelve hair-thin needles are inserted at specific acupoints in the body which stimulate channels of energy. The needles may be inserted for anything up to half an hour at a time. This releases the blocked energy at the acupoints, allowing the body/mind to relax, relieves pain and generally rebalances the body. Like acupressure, it also leads to improved circulation and stimulates blood tissues. Often acupuncture is often used in conjunction with osteopathy and kinesiology to guide and coordinate treatment.

Does it hurt?

Some who have tried acupuncture say they felt hardly anything at all. However, others say that some points can be painful or they may feel a slight pricking sensation, followed by numbness or a mild aching. This is said to be normal.

Who will benefit most?

Acupuncture can be used in the treatment of migraines, asthma, addictions, tennis elbow, paralysis, stroke, etc. In the United States acupuncture is the most frequently used alternative therapy for pain. The growing interest in alternative therapies has led some people to turn to acupuncture to help dogs and cats with arthritic conditions. People who use these services should make sure their vet is specially trained in acupuncture.

Is there any proof acupuncture works?

In the UK, the Home Office supports acupuncture in some of its prisons. During 2005 there was an outcry by victims of crime when acupuncture was used on some prisoners in order to relieve stress, alleviate depression and insomnia (Andalo 2005). Although there does not appear to be any scientific proof to support the claims by acupuncture therapists, the Home Office defended its decision as working towards a more holistic approach to medicine.

Are there different types of acupuncture?

There are several styles of acupuncture. However, they all work to the same basic principle of encouraging the flow of energy. The list includes:

- traditional Chinese Acupuncture: taught mainly in US acupuncture schools

- Japanese meridian acupuncture: uses thinner needles and gentler techniques

- Japanese Shonishin: specially designed for children, needles are not inserted but held or brushed over the acupuncture point

- Five Elements acupuncture: English approach to acupuncture which is based on European interpretations of classical Chinese acupuncture

- ear acupuncture (or auricular acupuncture): most often used for treating dyslexia and ADHD

- Korean hand acupuncture: uses needles to the hand only

- scalp acupuncture: uses points on the scalp

- cupping: a warmed glass or bamboo cup creates suction on the skin above a painful muscle or acupuncture point

- Emotional Freedom Technique (EFT): therapists tap with fingertips to stimulate meridian points

- moxibustion: a moxa (dried leaves) is burned in a cone above an acupuncture point to provide penetrating heat.

How many sessions are needed?

As with other alternative therapies, this varies from client to client. Usually clients are scheduled for ten to twelve treatments. Some advocates of acupuncture return regularly to keep themselves in condition.

Can acupuncture be dangerous?

Therapists claim that acupuncture presents very few risks. The tiny needles are sterile and disposable so there is no risk of infection. However, some clients report mild depression or anxiety.

Aromatherapy

Aromatic essences have been used for thousands of years (some records show their use in Chinese and Indian healing before 2000 BC) for their health-giving and mood-enhancing qualities. The French scientist Rene-Maurice Gattefosse looked at the healing qualities of essential oils and first termed the word aromatherapy. By the 1950s essential oils were being used on a regular basis.

Aromatherapy is classed as complementary healthcare, which means it works alongside orthodox medicine, and is one of the fastest growing complementary medicines in the UK and USA. Studies have shown that inhaling certain aromatic smells can bring almost immediate affect to the limbic area of the brain – the centre of our emotions and memory (Buck and Axel 1991; Wilkinson *et al.* 1999). The therapeutic power of essential oils helps the body to heal itself. Aromatherapy is a holistic treatment of the whole person, not just the symptom.

Approximately 400 essential oils are now used. They come from a wide variety of natural fragrant ingredients such as herbs, bark, flowers, petals, leaves, roots and the resin of trees. Some of the most popular are chamomile, rosemary, lavender and tea tree. Rosemary has been used for centuries in sick rooms. It works as a stimulant on the nervous system and where there is a reduction of function, including loss of smell, poor sight, painful muscles, etc.

According to research carried out by Dr Peter Warn (2004), some essential oils have been found to kill methicillin-resistant S. aureus (MRSA) bacteria and other bacteria. His study showed that three essential oils killed some bacteria after just two minutes of contact. The oils can easily be made into soaps and shampoos for use in hospitals. Researchers are seeking funding to continue their work.

How does it work?

At the first appointment the aromatherapist uses their skill to choose an oil (or blend several oils) to meet the client's needs and/or moods. All essential oils are diluted before use with a carrier oil such as olive, hazelnut or other 'soft' oils. The strength of the dilution is left to the aromatherapist to decide.

The client lies on a table whilst the aromatherapist combines the therapeutic effect of the essential oils with firm but gentle touch. Whilst the skin is being massaged the oils are inhaled and absorbed through the skin, directly into the bloodstream, resulting in a relaxed and harmonized individual. These benefits are said to continue long after the massage has finished. Essential oils can be used in a number of ways:

- inhalation – excellent for treating coughs or colds
- fragrant baths – a few drops of oil are said to be relaxing and relieve muscular pain
- compresses and hot poultices
- creams containing tea tree oil
- oils for massaging with the two senses of touch and smell having physical and mental benefits.

There are many different essential oils which are said to help with a variety of conditions including:

- mint for the relief of headaches and stress

- orange blossom as a relaxant

- lavender for hypertension

- ylang top for nervous tension and to inhibit frustration

- jasmine for listlessness and depression

- rosemary for stress disorders and to aid concentration.

It is said that an aromatherapy massage is one of the most relaxing soothing massages you can have. Clients who use it regularly say they are extremely relaxed and the effect lasts well after the length of treatment.

How many sessions are needed?

As with all alternative therapies length of treatment varies, but usually clients have three or four sessions to begin the practice and then decide to stop or come back on a regular basis.

Who will benefit most?

Many of us take flowers when we visit sick relatives. They look lovely, yes, but what we don't always realize is their therapeutic effect. A bouquet of jasmine, roses, geraniums and lavender contains chemicals that relax the nervous system. The aroma of these flowers quickly evaporates and penetrates the skin, entering the bloodstream and enabling relaxation.

Aromatherapy is reported to help a number of conditions, including anxiety, back pain, depression, fatigue, migraines, stress-related conditions and hyper-activity.

Can aromatherapy be dangerous?

There are a few things to remember with essential oils. First, they should never be ingested. Second, they should not usually be used on pregnant women. Third, it is said some oils can interfere with prescription drugs (high blood pressure). As with other alternative therapies, a doctor should be consulted before any treatment.

Reflexology

Reflexology is an ancient healing art dating back to Egypt in 2330 BC, where it is depicted on the Physician's Tomb in Saqqara. The American ear, nose and throat surgeon, Dr William Fitzgerald, introduced reflexology therapy to the west in 1913. During the 1930s Eunice Ingham refined and developed it further. Ingham found that congestion in any part of the foot mirrors congestion in a corresponding part of the body. Thus, by treating the big toe there is a related effect in the head, and treating the whole foot can have a relaxing and healing effect on the whole body. There are over 25,000 certified reflexologists registered worldwide.

In ancient times people walked barefoot over rocks, stones and other rough surfaces, which reflexologists believe naturally stimulated pressure points in the feet. Because of the way we live today, this natural stimulation has been lost. Reflexology helps to restore this balance and provide overall relaxation, rhythm and balance.

The science behind reflexology is based on the manipulation (massage) of pressure points, primarily in the feet. Applying pressure to the points that directly correspond to specific organs and muscles in the body creates a stimulus which readdresses the balance.

How does it work?

The client is fully clothed, with the exception of the feet and sits or lies on a table. The practitioner starts to apply targeted pressure to the reflex areas in the foot, thereby restoring balance to the body. The focus of pressure on the reflex points releases the blockages and restores the energy flow. Reflexologists work to improve several areas, including circulation, relaxation and self-healing.

Does it hurt?

Some clients say that reflexology is not just a foot massage and that the pressure applied can sometimes be uncomfortable. However, others find it very relaxing.

How many sessions are needed?

As with any alternative therapy, treatment time varies but clients usually have three or four sessions to start with and then re-evaluate. Some clients go back on a regular basis to keep themselves in tip-top condition.

Who will benefit most?

Reflexology can be used for anyone, young or old, and even babies. Parents naturally touch and massage babies as soon as they are born, thereby building up a wonderful rapport. Reflexologists say that because it is a natural therapy it promotes a sense of well-being and can help alleviate a number of conditions, including back pain, allergies, migraine, ear aches, stress and hyperactivity.

Are there different types of reflexology?

There are a number of types of reflexologists working on different areas of the body. However, they all work on the same principle to clear out energy blockages and aim to bring the body's energy flow back into balance. The list includes:

- foot reflexology (most well known)
- hand reflexology which is one of the easiest areas to work on with young children
- facial reflexology, a fairly new development in this field
- ear reflexology.

Reiki

Reiki originated in Tibet, but it grew in popularity in the mid-1800s, when a Japanese monk, Dr Mikao Usni, began teaching it. Reiki is the Japanese word for universal life energy: 'rei' is the universal transcendental spirit or essence and 'ki' is the vital life force energy. Reiki refers to the energy that flows through all living things. Reiki practitioners transfer this energy when laying the hands upon someone. They have learned to increase their energy to a higher vibrational level, so they can channel higher amounts of the life force energy. It is this energy that practitioners try to balance in their clients. Reiki is a gentle holistic form of healing by hands and is said to restore and balance energy, reduce stress and aid spiritual growth.

How does it work?

When having Reiki treatment, clients lie on a massage table with pillows under their head and knees (often soft relaxing music is playing). The therapists 'float' or gently put their hands over specific points on the body for a few minutes at a time. The therapist acts as a channel for the energy to flow through to the client, enabling the client's own body to heal itself. The therapist is only a channel for the energy because it is not his energy that passes through his hands but a universal energy which leaves the Reiki channel strengthened. Reiki works with the entire body's energy system, treating the whole of the body not just certain parts. It is said to be an excellent way to slow down and relieve stress. Reiki promotes a feeling of deep relaxation. Reiki is different from other massage therapies because the practitioner's hands remain still.

Who will benefit most?

Reiki is said to be a deeply relaxing experience. It may alleviate a number of conditions, including sciatica, asthma, migraine, backache, neck pain and dyslexia. It always leaves a sense of calm and well-being.

How many sessions are needed?

As with other alternative therapies, this varies from client to client. Reiki practitioners say that regular use leads to an increase in well-being and total relaxation. Some advocates of Reiki return regularly to keep themselves in balance.

Bowen Technique

The Bowen Technique was developed by Tom Bowen in Victoria, Australia. Like most alternative therapies the technique focuses on the body as a whole. This therapy makes use of the body's ability to heal itself through gentle 'rolling' movements on the skin. It is thought that this type of pressure on certain points realigns the energy in the body, bringing it back into harmony.

Bowen treatment claims to reset the body. Since we all have an ability to heal ourselves, it is useful for everyone from babies to the elderly. The technique is said to be particularly beneficial on sports injuries by activating the lymphatic system and combating swelling.

How does it work?

The client lies on a bed and the therapist works mainly on the client's back, legs and neck. Applying gentle pressure and a rolling movement, the therapist uses her fingers and thumbs across the muscles, tendons and ligaments. This action is said to disturb the muscle and create an energy surge, normalizing the body's energies. At regular intervals the therapist leaves the room and allows the client's body to relax.

How many sessions are needed?

Treatment usually lasts between half an hour to an hour and some clients go for regular treatments to keep their body in good balance. Clients report a very relaxed state.

Who will benefit most?

Bowen therapists claim excellent results with a wide range of disorders, including sporting injuries, allergies, cerebral palsy, asthma, dyslexia and ADHD.

Emotional Freedom Technique

In the 1980s Gary Craig refined the work of an American psychologist, Roger Callahan, to form what is now known as Emotional Freedom Technique (EFT). Craig worked to reduce the 300 pressure points to just 11, simplifying the whole area of EFT. This technique releases blocked energy patterns in the body and mind. Therapists say that emotional issues often clear quickly and easily. EFT is similar to acupressure, acupuncture, yoga and hypnotherapy.

What happens in treatment?

EFT works by stimulating acupressure points on the upper body, face or hands whilst focusing on specific issues. The patient remains fully clothed and the therapist uses the fingertips to 'tap' all 11 acupressure points. This in turn neutralizes disruptions in the body's electrical system and releases unseen blockages. The therapy is sometimes described as like acupuncture without using needles or any other implements.

How many sessions are needed?

Some patients will have one session with the therapist. Others find that once they have cleared their main problem different issues may arise and they return for further sessions.

Can this be done at home?

This therapy can easily be taught to the patient so he or she can practise at home. No equipment is necessary. There are training courses in over 56 countries worldwide.

Who will benefit most?

EFT therapists have good results with a range of conditions, including back pain, migraine, stress, frozen shoulder and dyslexia.

Summing up

'Rub it better' – my parents always used to say when you bumped yourself and I am sure many of us will have heard it, or indeed said it to our children. The mere touch of rubbing the place where it is sore automatically makes you feel better, probably because when you massage an area the blood rushes to that point to help repair the damage. Therapists tend to work specifically on targeted areas, using deep manipulation helping people with deep rooted scar tissue etc.

As with other therapies in this book they can be expensive but some have shown to be effective in just a few sessions. The best thing about massage therapy is you don't have to have something specifically wrong with you to go to a therapist. Going to an aromatherapist using different oils on you can be relaxing and is seen by many as a pure treat!

For useful addresses, please go to p.122.

Chapter 9

HOLISTIC HEALING

When looking for a therapy that can 'heal' naturally, there is a wide choice to consider. The therapies described in this chapter work in a holistic and natural way to promote good health, strengthen the immune system, help flush out toxins and provide stimulation and relaxation. Many of these therapists work alongside medical professionals and often doctors refer clients to them. There are a number of related 'touch therapies' with different methods to help you. The list includes:

- naturopathy
- homeopathy
- flower remedies
- crystals.

Naturopathy

Naturopathy promotes positive health by removing obstructions to vitality while supporting the body's inherent ability to heal itself. Full health can be achieved by optimizing the body's natural equilibrium with diet, exercise and fresh air.

How does it work?

Like many alternative therapies, naturopathy treats the whole person, taking into account their physical and emotional health. It is seen as a safe, quick and effective method of healing. Naturopathy calls on various alternative therapies to work together, thereby assisting the body to overcome illness by stimulating the natural defence processes from within. This treatment can be developed through various other alternative therapies, including:

- acupuncture

- aromatherapy

- herbalism

- nutrition

- hydrotherapy

- relaxation techniques.

It is claimed that naturopathy can help with hormonal inbalances, blood pressure, arthritis and many other conditions, including learning difficulties.

Homeopathy

Homeopathy is a complete natural treatment that encourages the body's healing processes to be self-regulating. It is a method of treatment based on nature's Law of Cure, namely 'Like cures like'. In 1796 Dr Samuel Hahnemann, a German scientist, claims to have discovered the truth of this law and spent his life working and developing these principles. Hahneman's work was developed further in 1877 by a professor of anatomy, James Tyler Kent, who worked at the American Medical College, St Louis. However, despite some people's belief in homeopathy, there is still a huge amount of controversy surrounding this issue with many people claiming that homeopathy is no different from a placebo. For a discussion of this issue, see Shang, Huwiler-Müntener, Nartey *et al.* 2005.

The principle of homeopathy can be seen in some parts of mainstream medicine, for example, antidotes and vaccines. Homeopathic remedies are said to be based on three principles:

1. 'Like cures like' – if the symptoms of your cold are similar to poisoning by mercury, then mercury would be your homeopathic remedy.

2. Minimal dose – extremely diluted form.

3. Single remedy – only one remedy is taken aimed at all your symptoms.

Homeopathy is said to be the second most widely used therapy in the world. After a slow start in the United States, the last decade has seen a growth of between 25 to 50% of people using it.

How does it work?

Like many alternative therapies, homeopathy treats the whole person, taking into account the person's physical and emotional health. It is seen as a safe, quick and effective method of healing. Homeopathy assists the body to overcome illness by stimulating the natural defence processes from within. There are over 2500 homeopathic medicines available made from a variety of sources, including vegetables, animals, minerals and chemicals. These remedies work by stimulating the body's own healing power. For instance, sometimes when you peel onions, your eyes may stream. This is the same symptom as hay fever sufferers have. If you then take the onion in its potentized form as a medicine, it can treat the symptom of hay fever. Homeopathic medicines are seen as safe because they are diluted to infinitesimally small amounts of the original form. Despite this very low dosage, the body responds well and can bring about a safe cure.

Homeopathic medicine is usually taken as pills, which are placed under the tongue, several times a day. These pills should not be touched by the skin (including fingers) but simply dropped onto the lid and put into the mouth. Occasionally some remedies are taken as an ointment and applied directly to the affected area.

Can homeopathic remedies help dyslexia?

Homeopathic remedies that are said specifically to help with ADHD are stramonium, cina and hyoscyamus niger. Pulsatilla is also said to help people with dyslexia.

How many sessions are needed?

Sometimes it may take a few visits to the homeopath to get the correct remedy.

Guide to self-diagnosis

ABC of Homeopathy offers a free online homeopathic remedy finder, making it easy to narrow down the choice of remedies for first aid and disease from the home (see Useful addresses).

Flower remedies

For centuries people have been using plants and flowers as medicine. Flower remedies use the essences of flowers to help alleviate emotional and stress-related conditions. The best known flower remedies are those by Dr Edward Bach (pronounced 'batch') who is considered to be the 'father' of modern flower essences. During the 1930s when Bach was practising medicine in Harley Street, London, he became convinced that many illnesses had their roots in mental and emotional states.

He sought an alternative to curing a patient's physical symptoms with conventional medicine.

Bach classified people's different moods into seven categories and then subdivided these into 38 negative feelings. He set about experimenting with flowers, plants and shrubs to see how they could affect mood. Then through a process of trial and error (and many years of patience) he was able to identify 38 flower essences that he considered could improve these negative feelings. This development became known as Bach Flower Remedies.

During the 1970s, further flower essences were developed by the American Richard Katz and since then other essences have been identified. Flower remedies can be used on their own but are often part of other therapies.

How does it work?

Flower remedies are usually referred to as holistic medicine because, as with other alternative therapies, the person is looked at as a whole, whereas in traditional medicine only the symptoms are considered. Therapists will take a careful history and then select a combination of up to seven remedies required for treatment, thereby ensuring every flower remedy is unique.

How are flower essences made?

Flower essences are made by putting flowers into spring water in the sun. This makes a solution filled with the essences of the flowers and the energy of the sun. Only natural ingredients are used in Bach Flower Therapy. Whilst Bach often used brandy as a preservative, this is now usually replaced by ethyl alcohol. For people intolerant of alcohol, for whatever reason, this can be replaced with vinegar. The flower essences are usually taken orally, diluted many times with mineral water, although they are sometimes applied to the skin. In the United States, Bach Flower Remedies are FDA approved.

Can Bach Flower Remedies help dyslexia?

Flower remedies that are said to help specifically with dyslexia and other learning difficulties include California wild rose, dill, five-flower formula, arnica, star of Bethlehem, rosemary, shasta daisy, mariposa lily, chestnut bud, vervain, lavender, Indian pink, madia, angelica and yarrow.

How are flower essences sold?

Flower remedies are supplied in liquid or salve form. A few drops of the concentrated/lower essence are placed in mineral water which can then be sipped, put on the lips, behind the ears or on the wrists. The skin salve may be used on the hands and feet and is also helpful for babies' nappy rash.

Who will benefit most?

Bach Flower Remedies practitioners claim they are best used to treat a range of negative emotions, including anxiety, shock, panic attacks, and lack of self-confidence. Dyslexia, ADHD and other learning difficulties are understood to be helped by alleviating the symptoms, primarily of stress.

Are there different types of flower remedies?

There are a number of types of flower remedies available. However, they all work to the same principle and aim to bring the body back to a calm and relaxed state:

- Bach Flower Remedies (most well known)
- international flower remedies from California, Eastern and Western Australia and Alaska.

Do I need to see a therapist?

There is a useful 'starter' book which gives a good indication of what is on offer (*Introduction to the Benefits of the Bach Flower Remedies* by Jane Evans 1974). Decide what the therapy is for and then buy several different remedies to help. Many health shops also stock a range of the essences.

Crystals

Quartz crystals and gemstones have been used for magical rituals and as a source of personal energy and healing for centuries. Crystal healers believe that the powers of the earth's energies have been absorbed by crystals. These vital healing powers can be used for almost any type of condition. Crystal therapy is a healing modality that works directly with the light, colour, beauty and perfect geometric forms that the mineral kingdom provides to assist in balancing all aspects of our being. It is said to be an advanced healing art that has the capacity to influence the physical, mental, emotional and spiritual bodies.

How does it work?

There are many different crystals but they appear to work in similar ways. For instance, it is said that Sugilite (Luvulite) helps people with dyslexia by enhancing the function of the pineal pituitary and adrenal glands. This activates and balances brain hemispheres, thereby helping anyone with dyslexia, coordination problems and ADHD.

It is important to keep the crystal on you at all times, 24 hours a day, for at least the first three weeks. This is said to help the cleansing process to be initiated and completed. This is also a period of time where the blockages of energy that are causing the imbalance are removed. Specific stones are placed upon the chakras or spiritual energy centres of the body.

Which crystals may help with learning difficulties?

Many different crystals are claimed to help people with learning difficulties, including dyslexia/learning difficulties, ADHD, memory, self-confidence and relaxation:

- dyslexia: Sugilite (Luvulite), Tourmeline/Black, Agate/Picture

- ADD: Fluorite, Hour Glass Selenite, Selenite, Azurite

- learning difficulties: Flurite, Azurite

- memory: Agate (Fire), Yttrian Fluorite, Rhodonite

- self-confidence: Quartz (Rose), Variscite

- self-esteem: Citrine, Kunzite, Golden Calcite, Isis Crystal, Oregon Opal

- relaxation: Blue Lace Agate, Turquoise.

Summing up

What better way of curing a problem than healing through natural processes? Flower essences, homeopathy or naturopathy all use natural products to help strengthen the immune system, to stimulate and relax you.

Many people swear by the use of homeopathy but it is still often seen as a controversial issue. As with many things in this book, you have to decide for yourself. Some, like crystals and gems, are inexpensive and if you find they help give them a go! At the end of the day, you just want to feel better, so try some different things.

For useful addresses, please go to p.122.

Chapter 10

THERAPIES OF THE FUTURE

Over the next decade I anticipate that more research will be carried out on the following therapies:

- Clinical Hypnosis (hypnotherapy): some people have had good results with weight loss, biofeedback systems (which work on similar principles) and more recently with learning difficulties.

- Light and Colour Therapy: this therapy has come to prominence in relation to seasonal affective disorder (SAD).

- Dolphin Assisted Therapy: swimming with dolphins may alleviate depression and improve cognitive responses in children.

Clinical Hypnosis by Angie Lawrence

Hypnotherapy is a treatment involving self-hypnosis – the art of attaining a heightened state of awareness in which the subconscious mind (the memory bank, the emotional and motivational force) becomes predominant allowing for positive thought and healing.

Everything that happens in our lives is recorded in the subconscious, affecting the way we perceive life. Our personalities are created by internal self-perception (endogenous) and external–environmental (exogenous) forces. Through my work I have come to believe that the environment determines human behaviour. We are conditioned from birth, thus we are the total of all our past learning experiences.

The area of the brain that records information is linked to the conscious mind in such a way that an emotional 'trigger' will cause the body to react and thus produce an emotional response based on the information recorded. For example, a young child who has had a bad experience will have recorded a negative 'trigger', and every time this situation is repeated the feeling magnifies, eventually resulting in an unexplained 'fear' or 'dislike' or a complete mental shutdown.

Clinical hypnosis is utilized to benefit the individual by using the powers of the mind to offer a solution, to heal and amend internal beliefs and perceptions to attain positive results. This may be attained by various methods and strategies depending on the needs of the individual.

The art of hypnosis can be traced back thousands of years, the oldest written recordings, 1552 years BC, may be found in the Ebers Papyrus. This document explained the medical practices of Egyptian physicians, methods still used to this day. Over the centuries hypnosis developed and in 1955 the British Medical Association approved hypnotherapy as a valid medical treatment, the US authorities followed suit in 1958.

Milton Erickson, an American psychiatrist and psychologist, is recognized as one of the most important contributors to the acceptance and use of hypnosis as a psychiatric therapy. He believed that clients could absorb new ways of thinking and learning without being aware that they are learning.

Hypno-Tech

This leads me on to Hypno-Tech, a technique for accelerated learning to remove negativity and build confidence and self-esteem through the use of suggestion. This method is designed to appeal to and tap into the subconscious mind of the learner through the use of hypnosis. Confidence and motivation have key roles to play in achieving goals and whether one is on the sport's field, on stage or in a learning environment the level of performance is determined by self-belief.

Hypno-Tech is a technique that helps organize the internal thought processes, to reassess self-identity to feel more comfortable in achieving attainable goals. Second, a learning environment is created that appeals to both sides of the brain.

RELAXED LEARNING – ABSENCE OF TENSION

When learners are relaxed and feeling good they can absorb and memorize facts more easily.

UNITY OF THE CONSCIOUS AND THE SUBCONSCIOUS, A RELAXED STATE OF MIND (HYPNOSIS)

Both sides of the brain are stimulated during learning, i.e. using the conscious reactions and functions while activating the subconscious to 'fix' the learning material.

GOOD RAPPORT BETWEEN INDIVIDUAL AND THERAPIST/TEACHER

The level of suggestive link (rapport) can be measured by how much information the student is absorbing. When the conditions are right, more knowledge is attained for longer periods of time.

These main features are important factors used in a hypnotherapy session yet may be incorporated into a learning environment provided Hypno-Tech principles are adopted.

Light and Colour Therapy

Light is the purest healing force in the universe. Pure white sunlight contains all the elements necessary to keep every living thing in perfect health. Just as we need a balanced diet if we are to be healthy, so also do we need a balance of all the colour vibrations in sunlight to nourish us energetically.

For centuries, people have been using different colours in their everyday lives. Most of us are aware that different colours evoke different responses. Vibrant reds are considered to be stimulating, whereas cool blues are soothing and relaxing. Studies such as Schauss 1979 suggest that colour influences moods, emotions and behaviours.

Light and Colour Therapy is based on the theory that light acts on the molecules of the body as a stimulative current. Coloured light travels through our eyes and triggers hormone production, which influences our entire complex biochemical system. Whilst some may think that this is a new age therapy, most people are not aware that light therapy is often used on babies born prematurely with jaundice. Until the 1960s some premature babies died or needed blood transfusions but now jaundice is regularly helped and treated by exposure to full spectrum or blue light.

How does it work?

Colour therapists help people to understand why certain colours are needed in their lives. They teach people how to use colours effectively – to heal, relax and inspire us. Colour practitioners claim that colour balances energy, aids creativity and learning and assists physical, emotional and mental conditions. They use colours and light for their healing abilities in treating emotional and physical problems.

Practitioners claim that sometimes just a quick change of clothes or a 'lick of paint' in the home or office can help people by relaxing or stimulating them (whichever is the desired effect) and, more importantly, can stave off depression.

By working on the colours that are supposed to either stimulate or relax, light therapies can be used in several different ways, including:

- colour light therapy – by selecting colours to wear, paint or change décor, etc.

- light or phototherapy – mixed colours, sometimes from a laser shone on a particular area of the body (or all over)

- ocular light therapy – light projected through coloured filters into the eyes

- colour reflexology and colour aromatherapy – two therapies used together.

Who will benefit most?

Some people have found that using light therapy such as a lightbox has been helpful to children with dyslexia and specific learning difficulties. Many dyslexia sufferers are also helped to read better with tinted glasses or overlays (see Chapter 6).

Colour therapists say that colour therapy can be helpful for various conditions, including seasonal affective disorder (SAD), asthma, bronchitis, dyslexia, ADHD and specific learning difficulties.

Can it be dangerous?

Colour therapy is often seen as harmless and is usually tolerated in most people. Obviously, exposure to bright light can cause injury and strobe lights may cause seizures in susceptible individuals. It is usually advisable to see your doctor before use.

Do I need to see a therapist?

Most clients usually see a therapist in the first instance and can then 'top up' at home. Some of the therapists loan the machines for home use. Otherwise machines are readily available now from several different companies.

Dolphin Assisted Therapy

For centuries dolphins have been seen as beneficial to the human race. In the early 1970s Dr Betsy Smith, an educational anthropologist, noticed the benefits of dolphins on disabled people. Whilst swimming with a group of dolphins, Smith noticed behavioural changes in both the dolphins and her severely disabled brother. She became convinced that dolphins could help people with a wide range of disabilities and developed Dolphin Assisted Therapy (DAT).

Dolphin Assisted Therapy was originally dismissed as a 'new age wonder'. However, in more recent years there has been a growing acceptance of DAT and it is now established in several countries.

How does it work?

Dolphin Assisted Therapy works by encouraging behavioural changes in people, partly using the method of 'positive reward'. Children usually spend half the session on 'floating platforms' in the sea and work with a trainer. The child helps to feed the dolphins and other small associated tasks. This work helps to develop patience, concentration, thought and coordination skills.

The second part of the session involves swimming with the dolphins. The dolphins are 'free' to stay and 'play' with the child or leave. This is said to help the child develop a number of social skills, including patience and relaxation. Equally, if the dolphin stays and 'plays' the child is rewarded with feelings of love and satisfaction. The therapy helps to increase thinking ability, self-esteem and improvement in communication skills. The child is encouraged to develop the motivation to participate, learn and think.

Children using Dolphin Assisted Therapy may improve in confidence and self-esteem and show a decrease in stress.

Who will benefit most?

Dolphin Assisted Therapy is said to help a variety of learning difficulties and alleviate symptoms of depression, post-traumatic stress and autism.

Summing up

Over the next decade, I believe we will see a huge growth in people trying to 'cure' themselves by going 'back to nature'. Hypnotherapy has seen a surge in popularity over the last decade; probably because a lot of television shows have shown how people can be made to do silly things. Therefore, if we take this to the next logical conclusion, it stands to reason that some of these actions could be used to reinforce good ideas, for example, weight loss or stopping smoking, or in my own personal case, to cure me of stage fright while singing.

However, in the case of the dolphins, I personally cannot see any ethical reason why we should allow these beautiful creatures to be used in this way. I am sure many people will say how dolphins have helped them, but I am sure some other alternative could be found instead of exploiting them in this way. For useful addresses, please go to p.122.

Chapter 11

BIOENERGY THERAPIES

Everything in the universe consists of energy. Quantum physics has revealed that we are energetic beings living in a world of energy. In energy healing human energy is known as bioenergy. Bioenergy therapies have their roots in traditional Chinese medicine, Applied Kinesiology and clinical psychology. The theory behind bioenergy healing is that the cause of all negative emotions is a disruption in the body's energy system. If the blockages are removed then the free flow of energy heals the body.

Bioenergy therapists believe that energy fields control how we feel from day to day and if the 'energy' is out of balance we may feel unwell. Work on the energy channels can rebalance the body and instil an inborn sense of calm, control and vigour. Bioenergy therapists believe that all creatures have an energy field (or aura) around them.

Bioenergy healing may sound new age but it is one of the oldest therapies around. In the east it has been believed for centuries that there are energy fields in and around the body.

Bioenergy therapists claim a wide range of conditions can be helped, including back-ache, breathing disorders, autism and dyslexia. There are may websites on bioenergy healing and its application for a number of conditions, including physical ones.

Can bioenergy healing be dangerous?

Most bioenergy healers will not treat pregnant women, people with heart disease and pacemakers and a few other health problems. It is always best to discuss medical conditions when asking about treatments.

Are there different types of energy healers?

There are number of related energy therapies with different methods, including:

- Bi-Aura therapy
- Electromagnetic Field (EMF) Balancing Technique
- Distant healing.

Bi-Aura therapy

Bi-Aura therapists are trained to work on the energy levels within the body. They seek out and remove energy blockages from the body's energy field. Once the energy blockages are removed from the body full health is restored.

What happens in treatment?

Whilst all therapists work slightly differently, generally, you stand in a room, sometimes candlelit, and the therapist moves around you scanning your energy field. The therapist passes their hands over the patient and can detect from the energy field what areas of the body are unbalanced or unhealthy by the feeling of heat or pain in their hands. They usually do this without touching you. For instance, the therapist may 'feel' intense energy in the patient's neck and the patient may confirm that they do have a neck problem. Once the therapist has identified the areas to work on, they start moving their hands around the area. They do not usually touch the area at all. Patients say they experience an odd and not unpleasant sensation a bit like a magnetic pull. It feels as if something is pushing down on the part of the body that is being treated. Some people may experience 'pins and needles'. Most people say they feel relaxed and positive at the end of each session.

Whilst the therapist is working they channel positive energy in through one hand and negative energy away from the patient through the other hand. When the patient's energy level is balanced they soon return to good health.

How many sessions are needed?

As with any treatment time varies, but it would appear that people usually have three or four sessions.

Electromagnetic Field Balancing Technique

Electromagnetic Field (EMF) Balancing Technique is a relatively new system of energy treatment pioneered by an American energy worker, Peggy Phonix Dubro.

Although it is still relatively unknown, EMF is now available in over 60 countries. Like the other bioenergy therapies, the EMF Balancing Technique works on the vibration of energy in the body. Therapists believe that working on a particular area of energy in the body will improve feelings of peace, self-worth and inner wisdom.

What happens in treatment?

Patients are treated lying on a couch fully clothed and the therapist uses very gentle hand movements (not necessarily touching the person), sometimes up to two feet away. Whilst performing these actions the therapist reinforces 'spoken intents' to clear, reconnect and balance the electromagnetic fields. As with other bioenergy therapies, some therapists claim to help and/or alleviate dyslexia and can assist with physical injuries.

How many sessions are needed?

This therapy is usually carried out in four stages.

Distant healing

Some therapists in the bioenergy field claim to work using distant (also known as absent or remote) healing. The therapists state that if a patient's 'energy field' is disturbed it can be controlled by the mind. There are several different types of therapies involved. For instance, Dr Usui, who developed Reiki, also developed the distant healing technique. He called it 'The Photograph Technique' because he required a photograph of the person asking for his help. Once he was in possession of the photograph/image, he could visualize the person to be healed and perceive their energetic information and imbalances. He could then send the Reiki energy to cleanse and balance the patient's chakras and energy.

How does it work?

Distant healing in the bioenergy field is sent from a bioenergy therapist, who could live anywhere in the world, to a person who has requested their help. Therapists practising distant healing say the results are just as good as face to face contact with a patient.

Summing up

Everything in the universe consists of energy. Bioenergy therapists have their roots in traditional Chinese medicine, Applied Kinesiology and clinical psychology.

Many people have not heard of this type of healing but in the East it is one of the oldest known to mankind. Bioenergy therapists believe energy fields control how we feel from day to day, that we all have energy fields around us and if our energy is out of balance we feel unwell.

Some people are sceptical about therapists who state they can cure them without touching or even seeing the clients themselves. But as with many of the therapies in this book they may be worth trying.

For useful addresses, please go to p.122.

Chapter 12

STRESS MANAGEMENT

When someone is worried, anxious or hurried the body begins to feel tense. This is a completely natural reaction because the body is preparing for 'flight or fight'. When the emergency is over, an 'all clear signal' is given and the body relaxes and returns to its normal state. However, when the body is under constant tension this produces stress, which needs to be reduced in order to relax. When the body relaxes it is sending the 'all clear' signal to the brain.

If children's bodies are constantly under tension they could display many different symptoms, including sleep disturbance, increased or decreased appetite, headaches, stomach aches, poor concentration or irritability. Their immune systems could also be weakened, thereby making them more susceptible to colds and other infections. Children with dyslexia and other learning difficulties often feel under stress, especially when they are at school.

What is stress management?

There have been numerous research studies over the last two decades supporting the theory that dyslexics and other people with specific learning difficulties suffer from increased levels of stress as a result of the difficulties they experience in the learning environment (see, for example, Gilroy 1991; Miles and Varma 1995).

Whilst we cannot look at the subject of stress in depth in this book, we can look at some of the ways that can help children reduce their stress levels. This will have a beneficial effect on their lives and also on schoolwork. If children are more relaxed they are more susceptible to learning. There are many ways to reduce stress levels including:

- laughter
- playing

- deep breathing

- rest and sleep

- positive thinking

- pleasant images/mental vacation

- meditation

- exercise

- avoiding caffeine.

Laughter

This is one of the best ways to reduce stress levels. Some hospitals employ clowns to go into wards to cheer people up. Apparently laughter releases certain chemicals in the brain, which is why we feel happy for a while when we have had a good laugh or watched a comedy on the television.

Playing

Playing games, running around in the park, climbing trees or skipping all produce 'feel-good' factors.

Deep breathing

When a person is tense their breathing becomes shallow and quick, leading to lack of oxygen. As oxygen purifies the body it helps to produce energy, so out with the stale old breath and in with the new.

You can try deep breathing exercises almost anywhere, but if possible find a place to lie down. Place your hands on your stomach and begin breathing deeply and slowly. Fill your lungs as much as you can and hold for a few seconds. Then slowly let out the breath. Do this a few times a day for about five minutes. You will soon feel the benefit of it. This technique is beneficial to children, especially those with ADHD, as it helps them to focus.

Rest and sleep

Although most of us realize the necessity for adequate rest periods, many of us, for whatever reasons, do not get enough rest. Tired and run-down feelings are common in those under a lot of stress. Children with ADHD often do not sleep through the night and wake every few hours. Try to get them to take a 'cat-nap' or even just lie down, or take them for a walk in the fresh air.

Positive thinking

This definitely works for me. Look for the good things in life, not the bad things, and you will soon find your outlook is changing. Every time you think something negative, make a conscious effort to change that thought into something positive.

Pleasant images/mental vacation

Children are particularly good at this enjoyable exercise (once they get the hang of it). Sit or lie somewhere comfortable. Close your eyes, relax your muscles and breathe slowly and deeply. Now try to imagine your favourite place. It could be the beach or the mountains or enjoying a favourite activity. Try to fully experience this imagined event. See the sights, hear the sounds, feel the air, smell the smells, look at the beautiful colours. Tune in to the sense of well-being.

Meditation

There are lots of different ways of doing this, but as far as I am aware they all use the basic principle of holding/slowing down the breath whilst focusing on an object of your choice and ignoring the thoughts and distractions around you. You could try focusing on a flower, a crystal or even fish in a fish tank.

Exercise

It is universally accepted that everyone should exercise three to five times a week for 20 minutes to keep fit and healthy. Walking is one of the easiest forms of exercise. Walk the children to school and back or perhaps have a football game after school. Walking is an excellent way to reduce stress and tension.

Caffeine

Some people think that caffeine is relaxing but it is actually a stimulant. It is much better to have a hot milky drink at bedtime.

CONCLUSION

There are over 50 alternative and complementary therapies in this book that claim to *help* dyslexia. Over the last 20 years I have observed that most children with learning difficulties suffer from very low self-esteem. However, with the correct teaching and the most appropriate CAM treatment I believe the symptoms of dyslexia can be alleviated. Many people (not even the specialists) do not know how these therapies work, but this is perhaps secondary to the fact that many have used these therapies and found them beneficial.

Having read this book, you could be forgiven for asking, 'With over 50 therapies on offer, what would you advise me to try first?' This is an impossible question for me to answer because it depends on the individual's problem. First, you have to identify exactly what type of problem the person has, for example, hearing or vision. Another important consideration is the personal preference of the person undergoing therapy. Which approaches fit in most effectively with their life and which tie in with their own comfort zones?

Some of the approaches have been included here for their relaxing effects and the way their alleviate stress. Others target problems that relate more specifically to dyslexia and specific learning difficulties.

When considering any of the approaches listed in this book, it is healthy to maintain a critical faculty, and to question what you are told, but equally make sure this does not prevent you from being open to some of the valuable treatments that are out there. By reading this book, you are in possession of information that can only benefit you and your family, so choose wisely. I wish you all the very best of luck.

RESOURCES

Books

Andalo, D. (2005) Guardian Unlimited Politics Special Reports, 2 June.

Andrew, S. and Chivers, M. (eds) (1996) *The Inner Hurt*. Peterborough: Poetry Now.

Barlow, W. (2001) *The Alexander Principle*. London: Orion Publishing Group Ltd.

Bérard, G. (2000) *Hearing Equals Behaviour*. New Canaan, CT: Keats.

Blythe, S.G. (2005) 'Releasing educational potential through movement: a summary of individual studies carried out using INPP test battery and developmental exercise programme for use with schools with children with special needs.' *Child Care in Practice 11*, 4, 415–432.

Bruner, A.B., Joffe, A., Duggan, A.K., Casella, J.F. and Brandt, J. (1996) 'Randomised study of cognitive effects of iron supplementation in non-anaemic iron-deficient adolescent girls.' *Lancet 348*, 9033, 992–996.

Buck, L. and Axel, R. (1991) 'Odorant receptors and the organization of the olfactory system.' *Cell 65*, 175–187.

Burgess, J.R., Stevens, L., Zhang, W. and Peck, L. (2000) 'Long-chain polyunsaturated fatty acids in children with attention-deficit hyperactivity disorder.' *American Journal of Clinical Nutrition 71*, 1, 327S–330S.

Butterworth, B. (2005) 'Developmental dyscalculia.' In Campbell, J.I.D. (ed.) *Handbook of Mathematical Cognition*. Hove: Psychology Press, 455–467.

Chinn, S.J. and Ashcroft, J.R. (1998) *Mathematics for Dyslexics: a teaching handbook* (2nd edn). New Jersey: Whurr.

Chinn, S.J. (1996) *What to Do When You Can't Learn the Times Tables*. Hertfordshire: Egon Publishers Ltd.

Chinn, S.J. (1999) *What to Do When You Can't Add and Subtract*. Hertfordshire: Egon Publishers Ltd.

Chivers, M. (1997) *A Parent's Guide to Dyslexia and Other Learning Difficulties*. Peterborough: Need2Know.

Chivers, M. (2004) *Dyslexia and Other Learning Difficulties: A Parent's Guide*. Peterborough: Need2Know.

Colquhoun, I. and Bunday, S. (1981) 'A lack of essential fatty acids as a possible cause of hyperactivity in children.' *Medical Hypotheses 7*, 673–679.

Dennison, P.E. and Dennison, G. (1992) *Brain Gym®: Simple Activities for Whole Brain Learning.* Venture, CA: Edu-Kinesthetics.

Dewhurst, R.J., Fisher, W.J., Tweed, J.K.S. and Wilkins, R.J. (2003) 'Comparison of grass and legume silages for milk production. Production responses with different levels of concentrate.' *Journal of Dairy Science 86,* 2598–2611.

Dyslexia Association of Ireland (DAI) (2005) Alternative Therapies Section. www.dyslexia.ie/alter.htm

Eden, G.F., Stein, J.F., Wood, M.H. *et al.* 'Verbal and visual problems in reading disability.' *Journal of Learning Disabilities 28,* 272–290.

Ernst, E. and White, A. (2000) 'The BBC survey of complementary medicine use in the UK.' *Complementary Therapies in Medicine 8,* 1, 32–36.

Evans, J. (1974) *Introduction to the Benefits of the Bach Flower Remedies.* Essex: C W Daniel Co. Ltd.

Garlick, D. (1990) *The Lost Sixth Sense: A Medical Scientist Looks at the Alexander Technique.* Sydney: The University of New Wales.

Gilroy, D.E. (1991) *Dyslexia and Higher Education.* Bangor: University of Wales Dyslexia Unit.

Grant, A.C.G., Howard, J.M. and Davies, S. (1988) 'Zinc deficiency in children with dyslexia: concentration of zinc and other minerals in sweat and hair.' *British Medical Journal 296,* 607–609.

Grauberg, E. (1998) *Elementary Mathematics and Language Difficulties.* New Jersey: Whurr.

Henderson, A. (1998) *Maths for the Dyslexic.* London: David Fulton.

Henderson, A. and Miles, E. (2001) *Basic Topics in Mathematics.* New Jersey: Whurr.

Hultquist, A.M. (2006) *An Introduction to Dyslexia for Parents and Professionals.* London: Jessica Kingsley Publishers.

Jordan, I. (2002) *Visual Dyslexia – A Guide for Parents and Teachers.* Brigg: Desktop Publications.

Koester, C. and Sherwood, B. (2001) 'The effect of Brain Gym® on reading abilities.' *Brain Gym® Journal 15,* 1–2.

Konofal, E., Lecendreux, M., Arnulf, I. and Mouren, M.-C. (2004) 'Iron deficiency in children with Attention Deficit Hyperactivity Disorder.' *Archives of Pediatrics and Adolescent Medicine 158,* 1113–1115.

Lyon, G.R. (undated) 'Why reading is not a natural process.' Covington, LA: Center for Development and Learning.

Madaule, P. (1993) *When Listening Comes Alive.* Norval, Ontario: Moulin, Appendix B, pp.191–192.

Miles, T.R. and Miles, E. (eds) (1992) *Dyslexia and Mathematics.* London: Routledge.

Miles, T.R. and Varma, V. (1995) *Dyslexia and Stress.* London: Whurr.

Morgan, E. and Klein, C. (2000) *The Dyslexic Adult in a Non-Dyslexic World.* London: Whurr.

National Research Council (1998) 'Preventing reading difficulties in young children.' Washington, DC: National Research Council.

National Reading Panel (undated) 'Teaching children to read: an evidence-based assessment of the scientific research literature on reading and its implications for reading instruction.' Bethesda, MD: National Institute of Child Health and Human Development.

Newby, M., Alridge, J., Sasse, Brother M., Harrison, S. and Coker, J. (1995) 'The dyslexics speak for themselves.' In Miles, T.R. and Varma, V. (eds) *Dyslexia and Stress.* London: Whurr.

Portwood, M. (2002) 'School-based trials of fatty acid supplements.' Paper presented at Education Conference, Durham County Council.

Richardson, A.J. (2002) 'Dyslexia, Dyspraxia and ADHD – Can Nutrition Help?' Paper presented at Education Conference, Durham County Council.

Richardson, A.J. and Montgomery, P. (2005) 'The Oxford–Durham study: a randomized controlled trial of dietary supplementation with fatty acids in children with developmental coordination disorder.' *Pediatrics 115*, 5, 1360–1366.

Richardson, A.J. and Puri, B.K. (2000) 'The potential role of fatty acids in attention deficit/hyperactivity disorder.' *Prostaglandins Leukotr. Essent. Fatty Acids 63*, 79–87.

Richardson, A.J. and Puri, B.K. (2002) 'A randomized double-blind, placebo-controlled study of the effects of supplementation with highly unsaturated fatty acids on ADHD-related symptoms in children with specific learning disabilities.' *Progress in Neuro-psychopharmacology and Biological Psychiatry 26*, 2, 233–9.

Schaffer, R.J., Jacokes, L.E., Cassily, J.F., Greenspan, S.I., Tuchman, R.F. and Stemmer Jr, P.J. (2001) 'Effect of Interactive Metronome® training on children with ADHD.' *American Journal of Occupational Therapy 2*, 155–162.

Schauss, A.G. (1979) 'Tranquilizing effect of colour reduces aggressive behaviour and potential violence.' *Journal of Orthomolecular Medicine, Psychiatry 8*, 4, 218–221.

Schulte-Körne, G., Deimel, W., Bartling, J. and Remschmidt, H. (1998) 'Auditory processing and dyslexia: evidence for a specific speech processing deficit.' Auditory and Vestibular Systems, Lateral Line. *Neuroreport 9*, 2, 337–340.

Shang, A. Huwiler-Mütener, K., Nartey, L., Jüni, P., Dörig, S., Sterne, J.A.C., Pewsner, D. and Egger, M. (2005) 'Are the clinical effects of homeopathy placebo effects? Comparative study of placebo-controlled trials of homeopathy and allopathy.' *The Lancet 366*, 9487, 762–732.

Tulip Financial Group (2003) Study commissioned by BBC2 for series *The Mind of a Millionaire.*

Warn, P. (2004) 'Essential oils could stamp out spread of MRSA.' Online article. Manchester: University of Manchester.

Wilkinson, S., Aldridge, J., Salmon, I., Cain, E. and Wilson, B. (1999) 'An evaluation of aromatherapy massage in palliative care.' *Palliative Medicine* 13, 5, 409–17.

CD

Butterworth, B. (2003) *Dyscalculia Screener.* London: nferNelson. (Software and manual)

DVDs

Darcey Bussell: Pilates for Life. (2006) Virgin.

Leah Bracknell – Yoga and You. (2003) Universal Pictures Video.

Pilates Body with Lynne Robinson. (2004) Firefly Entertainment.

The Alexander Technique – Discover Freedom from Stress. (2005)

The Alexander Technique – First Lesson and Solutions. (2000) Wellspring Media.

Yoga for Beginners. (2004) Prism Leisure Corporation.

Other

Belgau, F. and Belgau, B. (1982) *Learning Breakthrough Program.* Port Angeles, WA:
   Balametrics, Inc.

USEFUL ADDRESSES

General

Alternative therapies, dyslexia and SpLDs
Website dedicated to complementary and alternative therapies and Dyslexia/SpLDs.
Website: *www.alternativetherapiesdyslexia.com*

American Holistic Medical Association (AHMA)
12101 Menaul Blvd NE
Suite C
Albuquerque
NM 87112 USA
Tel: 001 505 292 7788
Website: *www.holisticmedicine.org*

AHMA is working towards transforming healthcare to integrate all aspects of well-being, including physical, environmental, mental, emotional, spiritual and social health; thereby contributing to the healing of ourselves and our planet.

British Complementary Medicine Association (BMCA)
PO Box 5122
Bournemouth BH8 0WG UK
Tel: 00 44 (0)845 345 5977
Website: *www.bcma.co.uk*

BCMA is the oldest organization representing therapists and has over 20,000 registered practitioners.

Complementary Medicine Association of Wales (Hypnotherapy Swansea)
12a Alexandra Road
Gorseinon
Swansea
West Glamorgan SA4 4NW UK
Tel: 0044 (0)1792 897059
Website: *www.hypnotherapy-swansea.co.uk*

Institute for Complementary Medicine (ICM)
PO Box 1941
London SE16 7QZ UK
Tel: 0044 (0)20 7237 5165
Website: *www.icmedicine.co.uk*

National Centre for Complementary and Alternative Medicine (NCCAM)
Bethesda
MA 20892 USA
Website: *www.nccam.nih.gov*

NCCAM is dedicated to exploring complementary and alternative healing practices in the context of rigorous science, training complementary and alternative medicine (CAM) researchers, and disseminating authoritative information to the public and professionals.

Natural Healing Institute of Ireland
Thompson House
McCurtain Street
Cork
Ireland
Tel: 00353 21 4501600
Website: *www.nhc.ie*

World Health Organization (WHO)
Headquarters
Avenue Appia 20
1211 Geneva 27
Switzerland
Tel: 0041 22 791 21 11
Website: *www.who.int*

WHO is the UN's agency for health.

Chapter 2: Identifying Learning Difficulties
Attention deficit hyperactivity disorder (ADHD)

Dyslexia A 2 Z (ADHD)
Website: *www.dyslexiaa2z.com*

Information on learning difficulties, ADHD, dyslexia, dyscalculia and other SpLDs.

Hyperactive Children's Support Group (HACSG)
Dept W
71 Whyke Lane
Chichester
West Sussex PO19 7PD UK
Website: *www.hacsg.org.uk*

Dyscalculia

Dyscalculia.org
8053 N. Delaney Rd
Henderson
MI 48841 USA
Tel: 001 313 582 6300
Website: *www.dyscalculia.org*

Dyslexia A 2 Z (Dyscalculia)
Website: *www.dyslexiaa2z.com*

Information on learning difficulties, dyscalculia, ADHD, dyslexia and other SpLDs.

Dysgraphia

Dyslexia A 2 Z (Dysgraphia)
Website: *www.dyslexiaa2z.com*

Information on learning difficulties, dysgraphia, dyscalculia, ADHD, dyslexia and other SpLDs.

National Handwriting Association
Website: *www.nha-handwriting.org.uk*

Dyslexia

British Dyslexia Association
98 London Road
Reading
Berkshire RG1 5AU UK
Tel: 0044 (0)118 966 8271
Website: *www.bda-dyslexia.org.uk*

Dyslexia A 2 Z
Website: *www.dyslexiaa2z.com*

Information on learning difficulties, dyslexia, dyscalculia, ADHD and other SpLDs.

Dyslexia Association of Ireland
Suffolk Chambers
1 Suffolk Street
Dublin 2
Ireland
Tel: 00353 01 6790275
Website: *www.dyslexia.ie*

Dyslexia Institute
Park House
Wick Road
Egham
Surrey TW20 0HH UK
Tel: 0044 (0)1784 222300
Website: *www.dyslexia-inst.org.uk*

Helen Arkell Dyslexia Centre
Frensham
Farnham
Surrey GU10 3BW UK
Tel: 0044 (0)1252 792400
Website: *www.arkellcentre.org.uk*

Dyspraxia

Dyslexia A 2 Z (Dyspraxia)
Website: *www.dyslexiaa2z.com*

Information on learning difficulties, dyspraxia, ADHD, dyslexia, dyscalculia and other SpLDs.

Dyspraxia Foundation
8 West Alley
Hitchin
Hertfordshire SG5 1EG UK
Tel: 0044 (0)1462 454986
Website: *www.dyspraxiafoundation.org.uk*

Chapter 3: Hearing

Auditory Integration Training (AIT)

Berard Auditory Integration Systems, Inc.
690 Boyd Rd
Leicester
NC 28748 USA
Tel: 001 828 683 6900
Website: *www.auditoryintegration.net*

Interactive Metronome®

Interactive Metronome®
2500 Weston Road
Suite 403
Weston
FL 33331 USA
Tel: 001 877 994 6776 (toll free); 001 954 385 4660
Website: *www.interactivemetronome.com*

Lexiphone

Lexiphone Technology Corporation
Website: *www.lexiphone.com*

Listening Centre (Lewes) Ltd
Maltings Studio
16a Station Street
Lewes
East Sussex BN7 2DB UK
Tel: 0044 (0)1273 474877
Website: *www.listeningcentre.co.uk*

Music therapy

British Society for Music Therapy (BSMT)
61 Church Hill Road
East Barnet
Hertfordshire EN4 8SY UK
Tel: 0044 (0)20 8441 6226
Website: *www.bsmt.org*

National Light & Sound Therapy Centre
80 Queen Elizabeth's Walk
London N16 5UQ UK
Tel: 0044 (0)20 8880 1269
Website: *www.light-and-sound.co.uk*

Sound Learning Centre
12 The Rise
Palmers Green
London N13 5LE UK
Tel: 0044 (0)20 8882 1060
Website: *www.thesoundlearningcentre.co.uk*

SAMONAS

SAMONAS
3435 Camino Del Rio South
Suite 336
San Diego
CA 92108 USA
Tel: 001 800 762 6627
Website: *www.samonas.com*

Tomatis

Tomatis Foundation Alfred A
Website: *www.tomatis.com*

Chapter 4: Bodyworks

Alexander technique

Alexander Technique Worldwide
Website: *www.alexandertechniqueworldwide.com*

Society of Teachers of the Alexander Technique (STAT)
1st Floor, Linton House
39–51 Highgate Road
London NW5 1RS UK
Tel: 0044 (0)845 230 7828
Website: *www.stat.org.uk*

Chiropractic

British Chiropractic Association
Blagrave House
17 Blagrave Street
Reading
Berkshire RG1 1QB UK
Tel: 0044 (0)118 950 5950
Website: *www.chiropractic-uk.co.uk*

International Chiropractors Association (ICA)
1110N Glebe Rd
STE 650
Arlington
VA 22201 USA
Tel: 001 800 423 4690
Website: *www.chiropractic.org*

Feldenkrais

Feldenkrais Guild
Tel: 0044 (0)7000 785 506
Website: *www.feldenkrais.co.uk*

Feldenkrais International Training Centre
PO Box 36
Hassocks
West Sussex BN6 8WZ UK
Website: *www.feldenkrais-itc.org*

Occupational Therapy (OT)

American Occupational Therapy Association
4720 Montgomery Lane
PO Box 31220
Bethesda
MD 20824–1220 USA
Tel: 001 301 652 2682
Website: *www.aota.org*

British Association of Occupational Therapists
106–114 Borough High Street
London SE1 1LB UK
Tel: 0044 (0)20 7357 6480
Website: *www.cot.org.uk*

Osteopathy

British College of Osteopathic Medicine
Frazer House
6 Netherhall Gardens
London NW3 5RR UK
Website: *www.bcom.ac.uk*

British School of Osteopathy (BSO)
275 Borough High Street
London SE1 1JE UK
Tel: 0044 (0)20 7407 0222
Website: *www.bso.ac.uk*

European School of Osteopathy
The Clinic
Boxley House
The Street
Boxley
Maidstone
Kent ME14 3DZ UK
Tel: 0870 412 8128 (UK) or Tel: 0044 (0)1622 671558 (INT)
Website: *www.eso.ac.uk*

Physiotherapy

Chartered Society of Physiotherapy (CSP)
14 Bedford Row
London WC1R 4ED UK
Tel: 0044 (0)20 7306 6666
Website: *www.csp.org.uk*

Pilates

Pilates Foundation UK Ltd
PO Box 36052
London SW16 1XQ UK
Tel: 0044 (0)7071 781 859
Website: *www.pilatesfoundation.com*

Pilates International
Unit 1
Broadbent Close
Highgate Village
London N6 5JG UK
Tel: 0044 (0)20 8348 1442
Website: *www.pilatesinternational.co.uk*

Yoga

British Wheel of Yoga (BWY)
25 Jermyn Street
Sleaford
Lincolnshire NG34 7RU UK
Tel: 0044 (0)1529 306851
Website: *www.bwy.org.uk*

Zero Balancing

Zero Balancing Association
Kings Contrivance Village Center
8640 Guilford Road
Suite 240
Columbia
MD 21046 USA
Tel: 001 410 381 8956
Website: *www.zerobalancing.com*

Chapter 5: Developmental Delay

Brain Gym ®

Brain Gym International
1575 Spinnaker Drive
Suite 204B
Ventura
CA 93001 USA
Tel: 001 800 356 2109
Website: *www.braingym.org/about.html*

EDU-K Foundation
12 Golders Rise
Hendon
London NW4 2HR UK
Tel: 0044 (0)20 8202 3141
Fax: 0044 (0)20 8202 3890
Website: *www.braingym.org*

Kinesiology Federation
PO Box 17153
Edinburgh EH11 3WQ UK
Tel: 0044 (0)870 011 3545
Website: *www.kinesiologyfederation.org*

Learning Breakthrough Program™
10 Sheldrake Lane
Palm Beach Gardens
FL 33418 USA
Tel: 001 888 853 2762
Website: *www.learningbreakthrough.com*
Orders: *www.learningbreakthrough.com/order.htm*

Primary Movement® (Martin McPhillips)
15 Ravenhill Road
Belfast BT6 8DN UK
Tel/Fax: 0044 (0)2890 222182 (04890 222182 from Republic of Ireland)
Website: *www.primarymovement.org*

Brushing technique

David Mulhall Centre
31 Webbs Road
London SW11 6RU UK
Tel: 0044 (0)20 7223 4321
Website: *www.davidmulhall.co.uk*

Chapter 6: Vision

British Association of Behavioural Optometrists (BABO)
Website: *www.babo.co.uk*

Keith Holland Optometrist
27 St George's Road
Cheltenham
Gloucester GL50 3DT UK
Tel: 0044 (0)1242 233500
Website: *www.keithholland.co.uk*

ChromaGen™

Cantor & Nissel Ltd
Market Place
Brackley
Northamptonshire NN13 7NN UK
Tel: 0044 (0)1280 702002
Website: *www.cantor-nissel.co.uk*

Coloured Overlays and Intuitive Colorimeter

Cerium Visual Technologies
Cerium Technology Park
Tenterden
Kent N30 7DE UK
Tel: 0044 (0)1580 765211
Website: *www.ceriumvistech.co.uk*

Harris Filters

Harris Foundation
Tel: 0044 (0)845 230 1771
Website: *www.harrisdyslexia.com*

Irlen Syndrome

Irlen Institute
Marita McGeady
14 Chalet Gardens
Lucan
Co. Dublin
Ireland
Tel: 00353 01 6280398
Website: *www.irlen.com*

Visual Tracking Magnifier (VTM)

Edward Marcus Ltd
Tel: 0044 (0)1226 764082
Website: *www.dyslexia.fsworld.co.uk*

Chapter 7: Nutrition and Health

Allergies

British Institute for Allergy and Environmental Therapy
Ffynnonwen
Llangwyryfon
Aberystwyth
Ceredigion SY23 4EY UK
Tel: 0044 (0)1974 241376
Website: *www.allergy.org.uk*

British Society for Allergy and Nutritional Medicine (BSAENM)
PO Box 7
Knighton
Powys LD7 2WF UK
Tel: 0044 (0)1547 550380
Website: *www.jnem.demon.co.uk*

Fatty acid supplements

(Efalex®) Efamol®
8 Brackenholme Business Park
Brackenholme
Selby
North Yorkshire YO8 6EL UK
Tel: 0044 (0)1757 633888
Website: *www.efamol.com*

(eye q®) Equazen
31 St Petersburgh Place
London W2 4LA UK
Tel: 0044 (0)20 7243 7100
Website: *www.equazen.com*

Herbalism

National Institute of Medical Herbalists (NIMH)
Elm House
54 Mary Arches Street
Exeter EX4 3BA UK
Tel: 0044 (0)1392 426022
Website: *www.nimh.org.uk*

Nutrition

British Nutrition Foundation
High Holborn House
52–54 High Holborn
London WC1V 6RQ UK
Tel: 0044 (0)20 7404 6504
Website: *www.nutrition.org.uk*

Feingold® Association of the United States
554 East Main Street
Suite 301
Riverhead
NY 11901 USA
Tel: 1 800 321 3287 (US only); 001 631 369 9340
Website: *www.Feingold.org*

Nutrition Society
10 Cambridge Court
210 Shepherds Bush Road
London W6 7NJ UK
Website: *www.nutritionsociety.org*

Chapter 8: The Power of Touch

Acupressure

Acupressure Institute
1533 Shattuck Ave
Berkeley
CA 94709 USA
Tel: 001 510 845 1059; 001 800 442 2232 (outside CA)
Website: *www.acupressure.com*

Acupuncture

British Acupuncture Council
63 Jeddo Road
London W12 9HQ UK
Tel: 0044 (0)20 8735 0400
Website: *www.acupuncture.org.uk*

British Medical Acupuncture Society (BMAS)
BMAS House
3 Winnington Court
Northwich
Cheshire CW8 1AQ UK
Tel: 0044 (0)1606 786782
Website: *www.medical-acupuncture.co.uk*

Medical doctors who also use acupuncture.

Aromatherapy

Aromatherapy Consortium
PO Box 6522
Desborough
Kettering
Northants NN14 2YX UK
Tel: 0044 (0)870 774 3477
Website: *www.aromatherapy-regulation.org.uk*

International Federation of Aromatherapists (IFA)
61–63 Churchfield Road
London W3 6AY UK
Tel: 0044 (0)20 8992 9605
Website: *www.ifaroma.org*

Bowen Technique

Bowen Therapists European Register
PO Box 2920
Stratford upon Avon
CV37 9ZL UK
Tel: 0044 (0)7986 008384
Website: *www.bowentherapists.com*

European College of the Bowen Studies
38 Portway
Frome
Somerset BA11 1QU UK
Tel: 0044 (0)1373 461873
Website: *www.thebowentechnique.com*

Emotional Freedom Technique (EFT)

Emotional Freedom Technique (EFT)
PO Box 269
Coulterville
CA 95311 USA
Website: *www.emofree.com*

Massage

Association Physical & Natural Therapists
27 Old Gloucester Street
London WC1N 3XX UK
Tel: 0044 (0)845 345 2345
Website: *www.apnt.org*

International Association of Infant Massage (IAIM)
88 Copse Hill
Harlow
Essex CM19 4PP UK
Tel: 0044 (0)7816 289788
Website: *www.iaim.org.uk*

Massage Therapy Institute of Great Britain (MTIGB)
PO Box 2726
London NW2 3NR UK
Tel: 0044 (0)20 8208 1607
Website: *www.cmhmassage.co.uk*

Reflexology

British Reflexology Association
Monks Orchard
Whitbourne
Worcester WR6 5RB UK
Tel: 0044 (0)1886 821207
Website: *www.britreflex.co.uk*

International Council of Reflexologists (ICR)
PO Box 78060
Westcliffe Postal Outlet
Hamilton
ON L9C 7N5
Canada
Tel: 001 905 387 8449
Website: *www.icr-reflexology.org*

Reiki

International Centre for Reiki Training
21421 Hilltop Street
Unit 28
Southfield
MI 48034 USA
Toll free: 001 800 332 8112
Website: *www.reiki.org*

UK Reiki Foundation
PO Box 1785
Andover
Hampshire SP11 OWB UK
Tel: 0044 (0)1264 773774
Website: *www.reikifed.co.uk*

Shiatsu

European Shiatsu School
High Banks
Lockeridge
Nr Marlborough
Wiltshire SN8 4EQ UK
Tel: 0044 (0)1672 513444
Website: *www.shiatsu.net*

Shiatsu International
Maulak Chambers
The Centre
High Street
Halstead
Essex CO9 2AJ UK
Tel: 0044 (0)1787 880005
Website: *www.shiatsu-international.com*

Shiatsu Society
Eastlands Court
St Peters Road
Rugby CV21 3QP UK
Tel: 0044 (0)845 130 4560
Website: *www.shiatsu.org*

Chapter 9: Holistic Healing
Crystals

Crystal and Healing Federation (CHF)
6 Buer Road
London SW6 4LA UK
Tel: 0044 (0)20 7736 0283
Website: *www.crystalandhealing.com*

International Association of Crystal Healing Therapists (IACHT)
PO Box 344
Manchester M60 2EZ UK
Tel: 0044 (0)1200 426061
Website: *www.iacht.co.uk*

Flower remedies

Edward Bach Centre
Mount Vernon
Bakers Lane
Brightwell-cum-Sotwell
Oxfordshire OX10 0PZ UK
Tel: 0044 (0)1491 834678
Website: *www.bachcentre.com*

Homeopathy

British Homeopathy Association (& Dental)
Hahnemann House
29 Park Street West
Luton LU1 3BE UK
Tel: 0044 (0)870 444 3950
Website: *www.trusthomeopathy.org*

Homeopathy Online Remedy Finder
Website: *www.abchomeopathy.com*

Society of Homeopaths
11 Brookfield
Duncan Close
Moulton Park
Northampton NN3 6WL UK
Tel: 0044 (0)845 450 6611
Website: *www.homeopathy-soh.org*

Naturopathy

General Council & Register of Naturopaths
Goswell House
2 Goswell Road
Street
Somerset BA16 0JG UK
Tel: 0044 (0)8707 456984
Website: *www.naturopathy.org.uk*

Chapter 10: Therapies of the Future

Dolphin Assisted Therapy (DAT)

Island Dolphin Care Center
150 Lorelane Place
Key Largo
FL 33037 USA
Tel: 001 305 451 5884
Website: *www.islanddolphincare.org*

Hypnotherapy

Angela Lawrence (Mind over Matter)
Mind over Matter
66 Pheasant Way
Cirencester
Glos GL7 1BL UK
Tel: 0044 (0)1285 652773
Website: *www.Mind-over-Matter.co.uk*

British Hypnotherapy Association
67 Upper Berkeley Street
London W1H 7QX UK
Tel: 0044 (0)20 7723 4443
Website: *www.hypnotherapy-association.org*

National Council for Hypnotherapy (NCH)
PO Box 421
Charwelton
Daventry NN11 1AS UK
Tel: 0044 (0)800 952 0545
Website: *www.hypnotherapists.org.uk*

Light and Colour Therapy

International Association of Colour (IAC)
46 Cottenham Road
Histon
Cambridge CB4 9ES UK
Tel: 0044 (0)1223 563403
Website: *www.iac-colour.co.uk*

SAD Lightbox Company
Unit 48
Marlow Road
Stokenchurch
High Wycombe
Bucks HP14 3QJ UK
Tel: 0044 (0)1494 484852
Website: *www.sad.uk.com*

Chapter 11: Bioenergy Therapies

Bioenergy Research Healing Foundation
4 Gloucester Road
North Harrow
London HA1 4PW UK
Tel: 0044 (0)845 456 1336
Website: *www.bioenergyhealing.org.uk*

Bi-Aura therapy

Bi-Aura Foundation
The Rookery
Newton
Northumberland NE43 7UN UK
Tel: 0044 (0)1661 844899
Website: *www.bi-aura.com*

Electromagnetic Field Balancing Technique

EMF Balancing Technique UK & Ireland
59 Windermere Avenue
Finchley
London N3 3RD UK
Tel: 0800 085 3765 (UK freephone); 0044 20 8349 1544 (international)
Website: *www.emfbalancingtechnique.co.uk*

LIST OF CONTRIBUTORS

Keith Holland, BSc, FCOptom, FCOVD, FAAO, DCLP

Keith Holland is an optometrist practising in Cheltenham, Gloucestershire, with a special interest in vision and learning. Over the last ten years he has built up one of the largest specialist practices in Europe, seeing children from some 44 countries, dealing with the visual problems associated with dyslexia and learning difficulties.

Keith has published many articles on the links between vision and literacy and lectures widely on the subject, both at home and abroad. He is the founder of the British Association of Behavioural Optometrists, a professional special interest group that represents practitioners around Britain working in this field. He is married and has four children.

Angie Lawrence, AMIH, CECCH, MNCH, MAPHP, GQHP

Angela Lawrence is a registered clinical hypnotherapist and psychotherapist practising in Gloucestershire. Her main clinics are in Cirencester and Cheltenham. Angela has been involved with psychotherapy for over seven years, specializing in Hypno-Birth and Hypno-Tech – a method she has devised for supporting people with learning difficulties. She has lectured at the Hornsby Dyslexia Centre in London to academics and parents on this special method of learning.

Angela is a member of the National Council of Hypnotherapy, the Association for Professional Hypnosis and Psychotherapy and registered with the General Hypnotherapy Register.

David Mulhall, BSc

David Mulhall is a leading expert in the field of neuro-physiological development. He specializes in treating learning difficulties and hearing problems across the spectrum of developmental delay. David trained at the Centre for Developmental Learning Difficulties and the Institute of Neuro-Physiological Psychology, Chester. He also trained with Dr Kjeld Johansen of Denmark, a pioneer in neuro-acoustic problems. The David Mulhall Centre opened in 1995.

Christopher Vickers, DC, MICS, FCC

Christopher Vickers chose chiropractic as a career after suffering a back injury at school; conventional therapy had not worked, where chiropractic had. He graduated from the Anglo-European College of Chiropractic in 1981. From, there he held an associateship in Edinburgh, followed by working in Zimbabwe and South Africa.

On returning to the UK in 1986, he became involved in learning about cranial work which he now teaches across Europe. During his work in this area he became increasingly interested in dyslexic problems amplified by having studied Neural Organization Technique (NOT). Christopher had a thriving private practice in Cirencester and is married with three children. He has recently emigrated to New Zealand.

SUBJECT INDEX

AUTHOR INDEX